The Wellness Chronicles

Book 33

Volume 5

By Jim Moltzan

Insights on Holistic Health, Wellness, and Ancient Wisdom

Physical & Mental Well-being:
- Societal & Ethical Health Perspectives
- Functional Anatomy
- Holistic Physiology
- Philosophy & Self-reflection
- Mind-Body Psychology
- Movement, Breath & Awareness

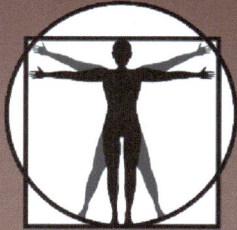

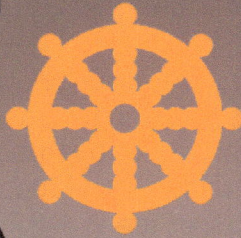

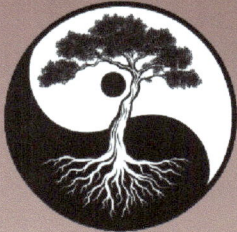

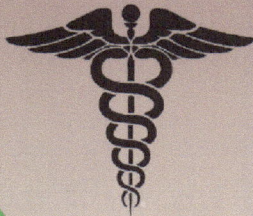

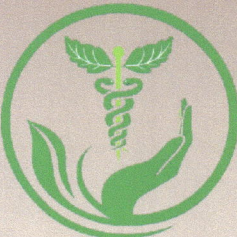

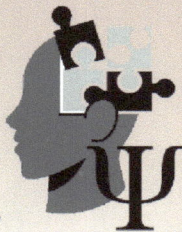

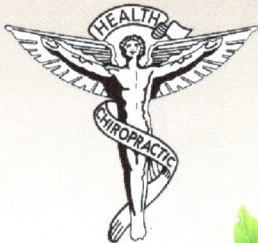

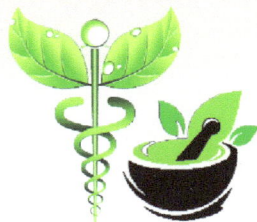

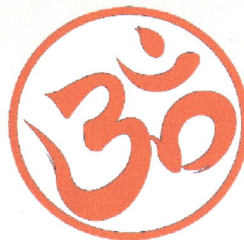

Disclaimer

This book is intended for information purposes only. The author does not promise or imply any results to those using this information, nor are they responsible for any adverse results brought about by the usage of the information contained herein. Use the information provided at your own risk. Furthermore, the author does not guarantee that the holder of this information will improve his or her health from the information contained herein.

The author of this book has used his/her best efforts in preparing this book. The author makes no representation of warranties with respect to the accuracy, applicability, or completeness of the contents of this book.

ISBN: 978-1-958837-43-6

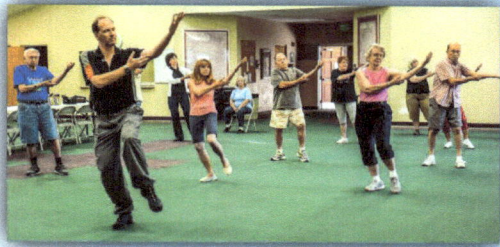
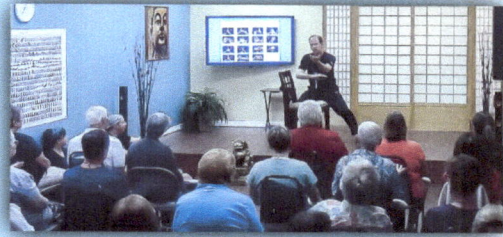
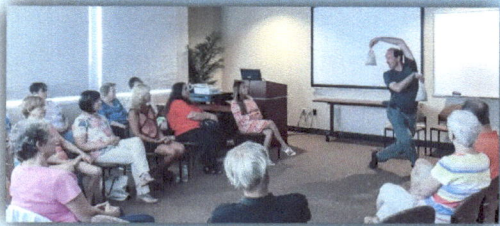
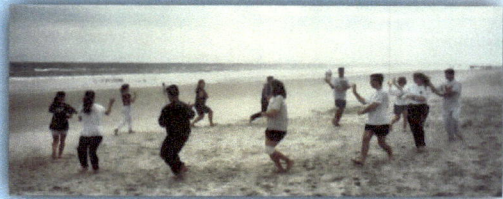
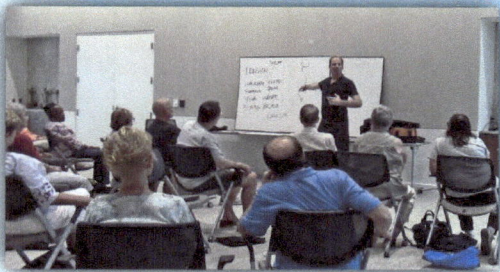
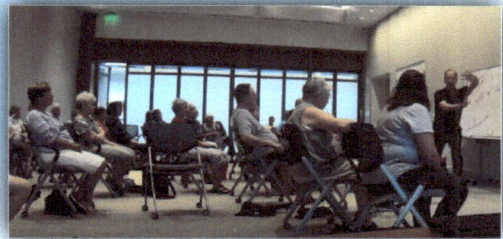
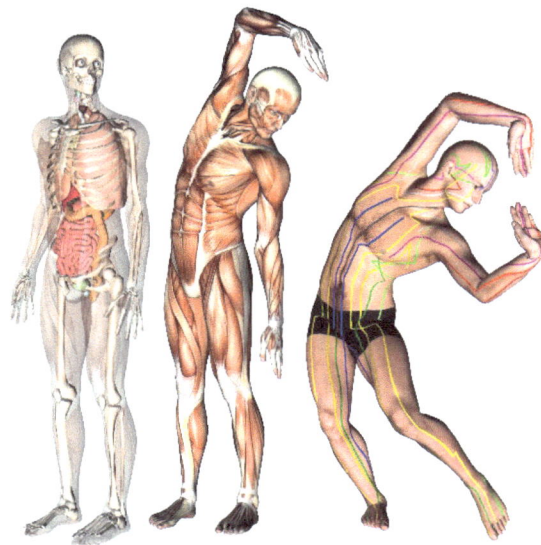

Foreword

The Wellness Chronicles: Volume 5 represents the continuing evolution of a lifelong commitment to holistic self-development of body, mind, and spirit. This work draws from over four decades of practice, teaching, and inquiry across disciplines such as Traditional Chinese Medicine, martial arts, breathwork, philosophy, and physiology. It is both reflective and practical, bridging ancient insights with modern challenges.

The articles and illustrations herein are not randomly compiled. Rather they are carefully organized into thematic sections that guide the reader through levels of awareness. I discuss topics from systemic health dysfunctions and cultural blind spots to personal responsibility, physical training, subtle energetics, and deeper consciousness. You will find discussions on government overreach and media distortion alongside Taoist cosmology, acupressure techniques, breath control, and the neurological power of balance and posture.

This book is neither a technical manual nor a self-help cliché. It is a record of insights earned through experience, struggle, practice, and contemplation. It is for seekers, skeptics, healers, warriors, and everyday people who want more than symptom management. It is for those who feel that health must include sovereignty, ethics, and connection.

Each section invites a new lens: societal critique, philosophical realignment, physical embodiment, energy restoration, emotional processing, breath cultivation, and neural integration. While eclectic in form, it is unified in its purpose to awaken awareness, personal agency, and a sustainable relationship with health.

Whether you skim a single essay or absorb the whole volume, may these chronicles remind you that wellness is not a trend, but a way of life.

With sincerity and purpose,

Jim Moltzan

Why I Share, What I Have Learned

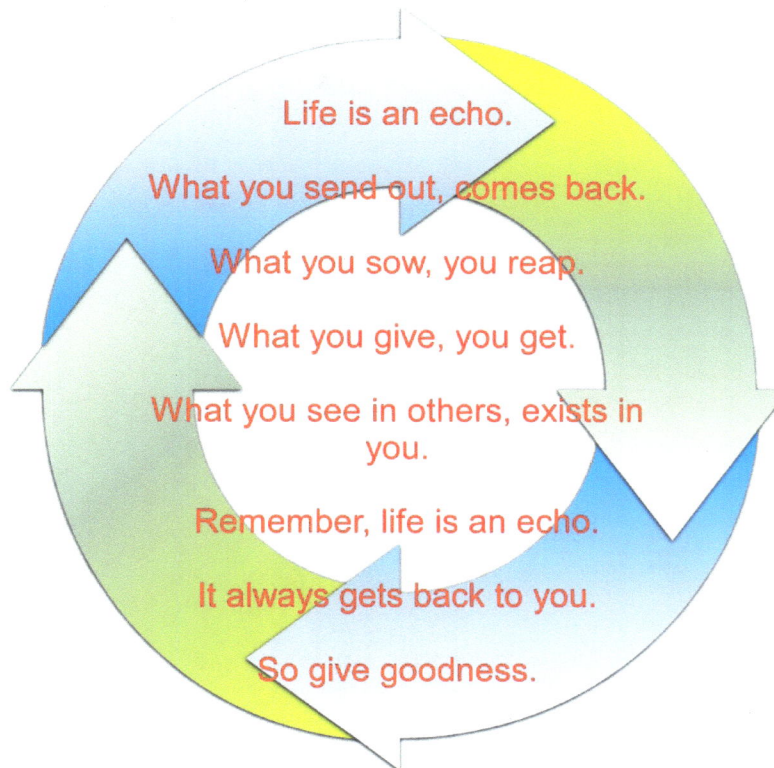

Life is an echo.

What you send out, comes back.

What you sow, you reap.

What you give, you get.

What you see in others, exists in you.

Remember, life is an echo.

It always gets back to you.

So give goodness.

www.MindAndBodyExercises.com

I made my commitment many years ago to learn, study, practice and teach fitness and well-being. My education came from martial arts and various other Eastern methods rooted in Traditional Chinese Medicine (TCM). I started when I was 16 years old and have never stopped since; 61 now.

I have written journals, produced educational graphics and co-authored a book in addition to many that I have self-authored. I blog often with a WordPress site, writing about the anatomical, physiological and mental benefits of mind and body training. Years back I started recording my classes and lectures, knowing that somewhere down the line, all of this information would be valuable to those who need and desire it.

My YouTube channel has almost 300 videos of FREE classes and other education videos. The goal all along has been to raise the awareness that Tai chi (a martial art), qigong (yoga at its root) and many other Eastern wellness methods, have proven the test of time for maintaining well-being. No gym, no mat, no membership, no special clothes or equipment. Just the individual and their engagement.

Weak or injured knees, back issues (strains & sciatica), stress & anxiety, asthma, arthritis, balance, poor posture - the list is endless. These are all issues that can be improved or overcome by those serious about learning about the mind, body & spirit connection.

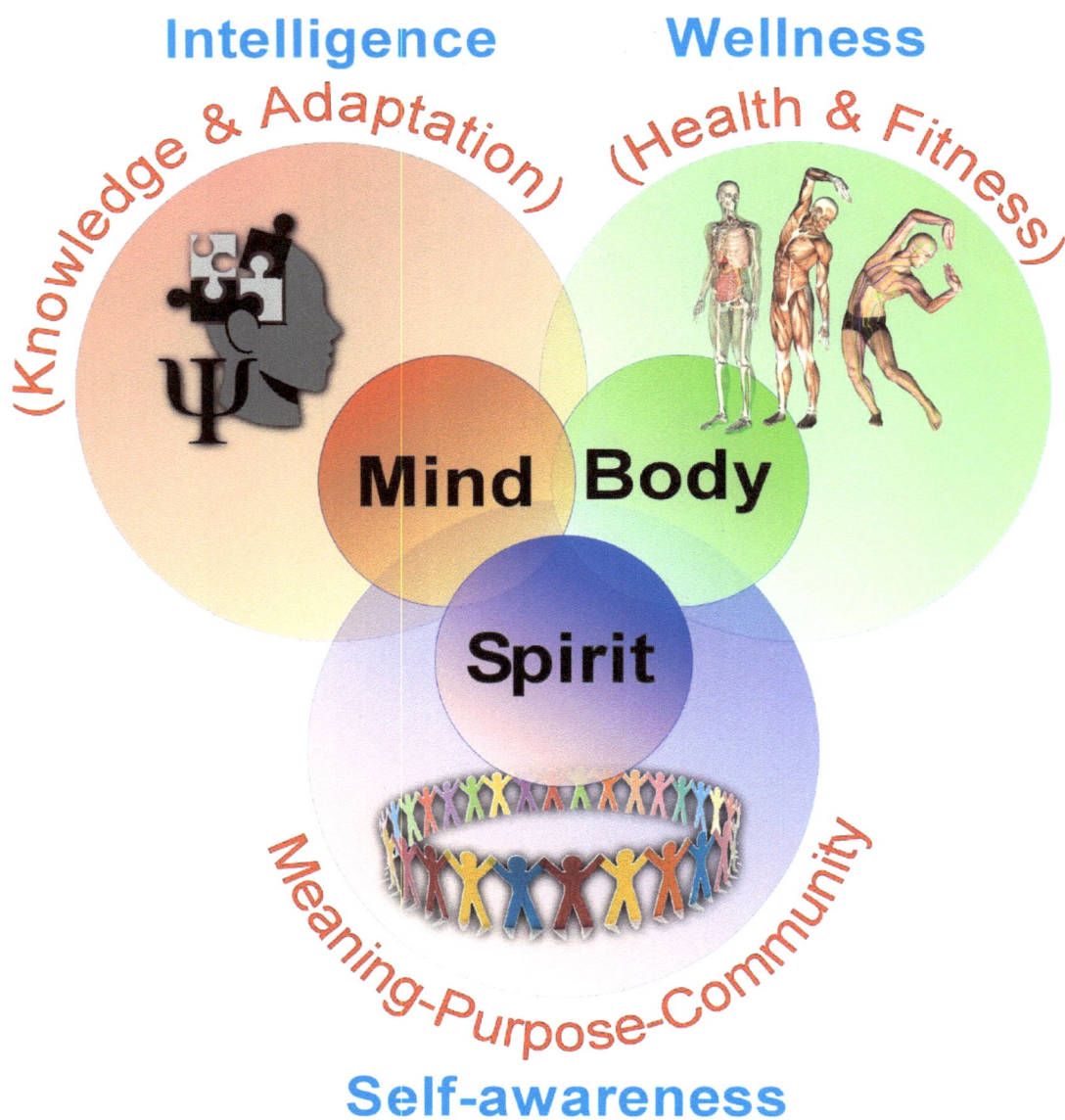

Intelligence

(Knowledge & Adaptation)

Wellness

(Health & Fitness)

Mind **Body**

Spirit

Meaning-Purpose-Community

Self-awareness

We are the architect of our own health, happiness, destiny, or fate.

Table of Contents

SECTION I: SOCIETY, ETHICS & HEALTHCARE SYSTEMS

Are Our "Protectors" Harming Us?

A Holistic Look at Government Dysfunction

In recent decades, there has been growing debate and public dissatisfaction surrounding the effectiveness of major U.S. government agencies such as the National Institutes of Health (NIH), Centers for Disease Control and Prevention (CDC), Food and Drug Administration (FDA), Environmental Protection Agency (EPA), and Department of Education (DOE). From a holistic health and wellness standpoint, the concerns raised are not only legitimate but crucial for the future well-being of American society.

Despite the enormous budgets allocated to these institutions, many key indicators of national health and environmental quality have not improved and in some cases, have greatly worsened. Rates of chronic diseases, such as obesity, diabetes, and autoimmune disorders, have surged over the past several decades (FaST FaCTs: Health and Economic Costs of Chronic Conditions, 2024). American food products are heavily processed and laden with additives, while issues such as polluted drinking water continue to affect vulnerable populations (Environmental Protection Agency [EPA], 2023). Meanwhile, the pharmaceutical industry's extensive influence over agencies like the FDA and CDC has raised serious ethical questions about regulatory capture and conflicts of interest (Abbott & Dukes, 2009).
The educational sector is similarly troubled. Despite increased federal involvement, American students have shown declining scores in key academic areas compared to previous generations (National Center for Education Statistics, 2024). From a systems thinking perspective central to holistic health, these problems are interconnected. Poor nutrition, environmental toxicity, and weakened educational outcomes contribute collectively to the degradation of overall societal wellness.

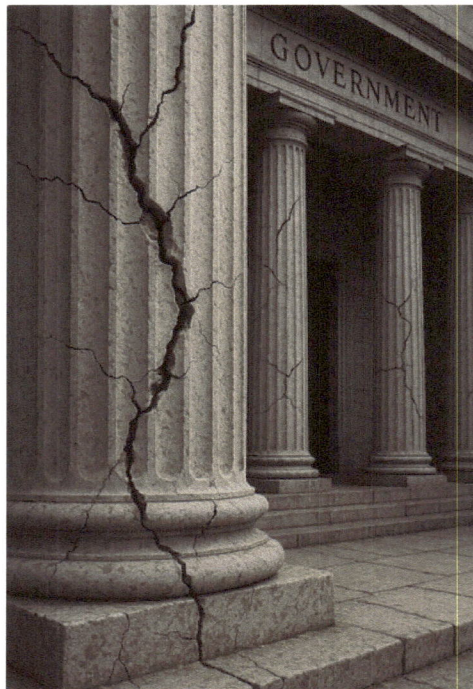

If these agencies operated within the private sector, the level of dysfunction witnessed would likely result in significant consequences for leadership, including firings, lawsuits, or even criminal prosecutions. Companies that consistently fail their customers typically lose credibility and cease to exist. However, because these government organizations are taxpayer-funded and politically shielded, they continue to operate with limited accountability. The principle of accountability is foundational to any healthy democracy. Citizens not only have the right but the *responsibility* to demand reforms when institutions fail to serve the public interest. As political theorist John Locke emphasized, government derives its legitimacy from the consent of the governed, and when it ceases to act for the public good, reform becomes necessary (Locke, 1988).

There is significant evidence that Americans are not being adequately protected or served in key areas of health, environment, and education, which are all pillars of a thriving and holistic society. It would therefore not be wrong, but entirely *appropriate and vital*, for citizens to call for drastic reforms or even overhauls of these agencies. From a holistic health perspective, reform is not simply a political preference; it is a matter of survival and future flourishing. Holistic wellness emphasizes balance, responsibility, interconnectedness, and long-term thinking. If the government institutions designed to protect health, the environment, and education are misaligned with these principles, it is imperative that we, as a society committed to holistic well-being, advocate transformative change. Without public awareness and pressure, the existing system will continue to perpetuate dysfunction to the detriment of both current and future generations.

References:

Abbott, F. M., & Dukes, G. (2009). *Global Pharmaceutical Policy*. https://doi.org/10.4337/9781849801843

Environmental Protection Agency. (2023). *Drinking water pollution and health risks*. https://www.epa.gov/ground-water-and-drinking-water

FaST FaCTs: Health and economic costs of chronic conditions. (2024, July 12). Chronic Disease. https://www.cdc.gov/chronic-disease/data-research/facts-stats/index.html

Locke, J. (1988). John Locke Two treatises of government. In *Cambridge University Press eBooks*. https://doi.org/10.1017/cbo9780511810268

National Center for Education Statistics. (2024). *The Nation's Report Card | NAEP*. https://nces.ed.gov/nationsreportcard/

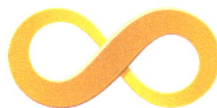

Global Affairs and Personal Responsibility

In studying world events, we often discover that things are not always as they appear on the surface. A powerful example of this is found in John Perkins' revealing book, *Confessions of an Economic Hit Man* (Perkins, 2004). Perkins shares his firsthand experiences of how the United States, through corporations, banks, and covert operations, orchestrated financial and political control over many developing nations, often in the name of "helping" them. According to Perkins (2004), the system worked as follows: economic consultants would persuade leaders of developing nations to accept massive loans for infrastructure projects. These loans, however, rarely benefited the local population. Instead, they flowed to large U.S. corporations like Bechtel, Halliburton, and Stone & Webster to build projects that made countries dependent rather than independent. When nations inevitably struggled to repay their debts, the U.S. could then leverage their vulnerability, gaining access to natural resources, securing military bases, or influencing critical political decisions (Perkins, 2004).

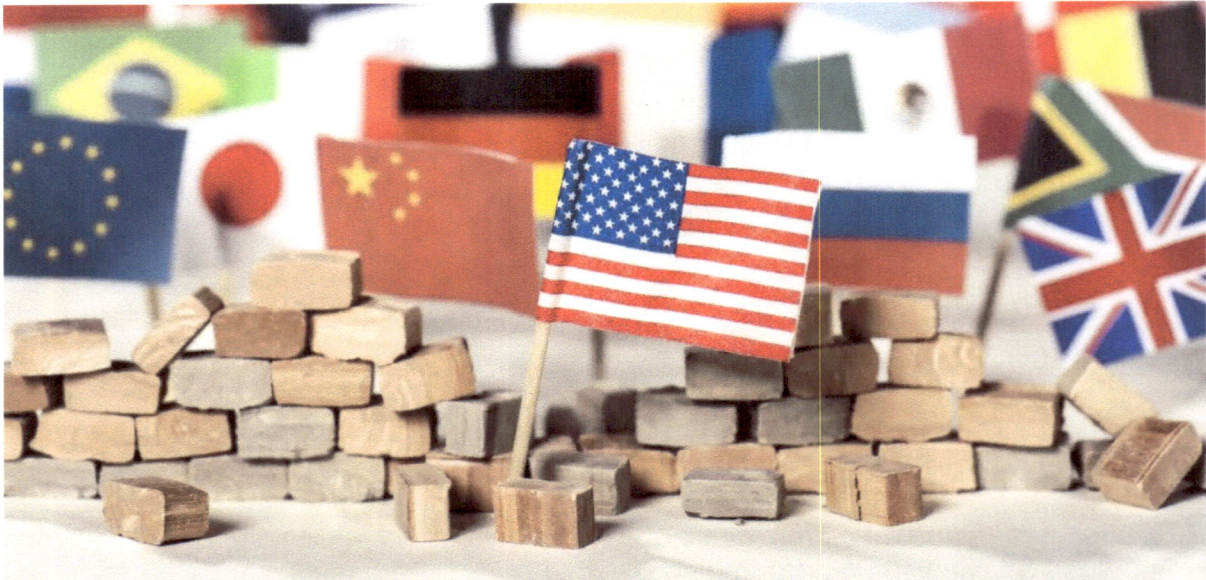

If leaders resisted, covert operations and sometimes violent regime changes would often follow. Historical cases such as the overthrow of Mohammad Mossadegh in Iran, the assassination of Omar Torrijos in Panama, and the toppling of Salvador Allende in Chile exemplify this pattern (Kinzer, 2007; Blum, 2003).

Institutions involved in this system included not just private corporations, but also public agencies like the World Bank, the International Monetary Fund (IMF), USAID, and even parts of the NSA and CIA (Perkins, 2004). While many Americans believed and still believe that their country acts as a global force for good, many people around the world have a very different perspective. For them, U.S. involvement often meant debt, exploitation, lost sovereignty, and prolonged suffering under authoritarian regimes supported by external powers (Blum, 2003).

What This Means for Our Own Lives

It's easy to become deeply engaged, even consumed by the pursuit of truth when uncovering these hidden histories. Indeed, understanding the deeper truths about global affairs can be empowering and necessary for conscious living. However, there is an essential balance we must maintain:

We must not let the pursuit of external truth eclipse the internal truth of caring for ourselves.

Chronic anger, outrage, and obsession can cause significant damage:
- Persistent stress weakens the immune system (Segerstrom & Miller, 2004).

- Excessive media consumption contributes to mental exhaustion and emotional burnout

- Neglect of physical well-being sleep, exercise, nutrition, etc. can diminish vitality and resilience.

In the end, truth-seeking should not come at the cost of self-care. When we are physically strong, mentally clear, and emotionally stable, we are in a far better position to discern information, resist manipulation, and lead by quiet example rather than reactive outrage.

A Healthier Path Forward

History will always be complex, layered with contradictions, hidden motives, and competing interests. Yet we do not serve ourselves or the greater good by burning out or losing our health in pursuit of endless investigation.
Instead, we can:

- Practice daily **mental hygiene**: mindfulness, conscious breathing, time away from media noise.

- Maintain **physical vitality**: nourishing the body through good food, movement, and rest.

- Build **emotional resilience**: cultivating gratitude, perspective, and compassionate boundaries.

By doing so, we remain rooted and strong and able to perceive global injustices without being consumed by them. Global interventions and economic manipulations have been supported by leaders from both major U.S. political parties. Historical evidence shows that Democratic and Republican administrations alike have engaged in coups, economic coercion, military interventions, and covert operations, often justified as protecting "freedom" or "democracy," but usually serving corporate and strategic interests.

Wellness means seeing clearly. Falling into the trap of blind loyalty to any party can cause mental fatigue, emotional burnout, and chronic frustration. True sovereignty begins with personal health and clear-minded observation, not blind allegiance.

Cultivate awareness. Stay grounded. Care for your own body, mind, and spirit first.

In conclusion, understanding global systems of influence can awaken us. But maintaining personal sovereignty of our own body, mind, and spirit is what ultimately allows us to thrive, think clearly, and live freely.

Awareness without health is a hollow victory.
Health without awareness is a shallow peace.
Both together create a life of strength, clarity, and purpose.

References:

Blum, W. (2003). *Killing hope* (By Zed Books London). Zed Books London. https://www.cia.gov/library/abbottabad-compound/13/130AEF1531746AAD6AC03EF59F91E1A1_Killing_Hope_Blum_William.pdf

Kinzer, S. (2007). *Overthrow: America's Century of Regime Change from Hawaii to Iraq.* Macmillan.

Lobe, J. (2024, April 26). What are Americans' biggest foreign policy priorities? *Responsible Statecraft.* https://responsiblestatecraft.org/us-foreign-policy-poll/

Perkins, J. (2004). *Confessions of an economic hit man.* Berrett-Koehler Publishers. Segerstrom, S. C., & Miller, G. E. (2004). Psychological stress and the human immune system: A meta-analytic study of 30 years of inquiry. *Psychological Bulletin*, 130(4), 601–630. https://doi.org/10.1037/0033-2909.130.4.601

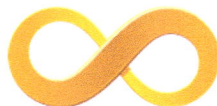

Spiritual Paradoxes: Humility Taught, Materialism Practiced

Across time and cultures, the greatest spiritual teachers have emphasized simplicity, humility, and inner transformation. Yet, paradoxically, the institutions that grow around these teachings often accumulate material wealth, political power, and ego-driven prestige. Christianity, Buddhism, Hinduism, Islam, all at their core, advocate for the shedding of worldly attachments. Yet many of their largest institutions exhibit the very materialism and hierarchy their founders warned against. In light of today's cultural unrest, consumerism, and spiritual seeking, these contradictions deserve closer reflection.

A Humble Beginning

Jesus of Nazareth lived with radical humility. His birth in a manger (Luke 2:7, New International Version [NIV]), his itinerant lifestyle (*"the Son of Man has no place to lay his head,"* Luke 9:58, NIV), and his repeated critiques of religious legalism (Matthew 23:1–28, NIV) demonstrate a clear rejection of material power and ritualized pretense. He warned against storing up treasures on earth, urging people instead to seek spiritual treasures (Matthew 6:19–21, NIV). His message was direct: inner transformation and compassion mattered more than public ritual or personal gain.

And yet, centuries later, the Roman Catholic Church emerged from the very empire that crucified him, to became one of the wealthiest and most ritualized institutions in human history (MacCulloch, 2011).

A Universal Paradox

This irony is not exclusive to Christianity. It is a universal pattern across major belief systems:

- **Buddhism**: Siddhartha Gautama, the Buddha, renounced his royal status to seek enlightenment through simplicity and meditation. His core teaching of the elimination of craving and attachment became institutionalized into monasteries and sects, some of which, over centuries, accumulated wealth, political influence, and hierarchical authority (Lopez, 2001).

- **Hinduism**: Early Vedic teachings stressed detachment from material life through paths like *Jnana* (knowledge) and *Bhakti* (devotion). Yet, sprawling temple complexes, priestly hierarchies, and caste structures often mirrored societal materialism and status-seeking (Flood, 1996).

- **Islam**: The Prophet Muhammad lived simply, called for humility, and emphasized equality among believers. Yet throughout history, caliphates and modern regimes alike have at times entangled faith with vast political and material ambitions (Esposito, 1998).

Again and again, humanity seems to be drawn to codify spiritual simplicity into worldly complexity.

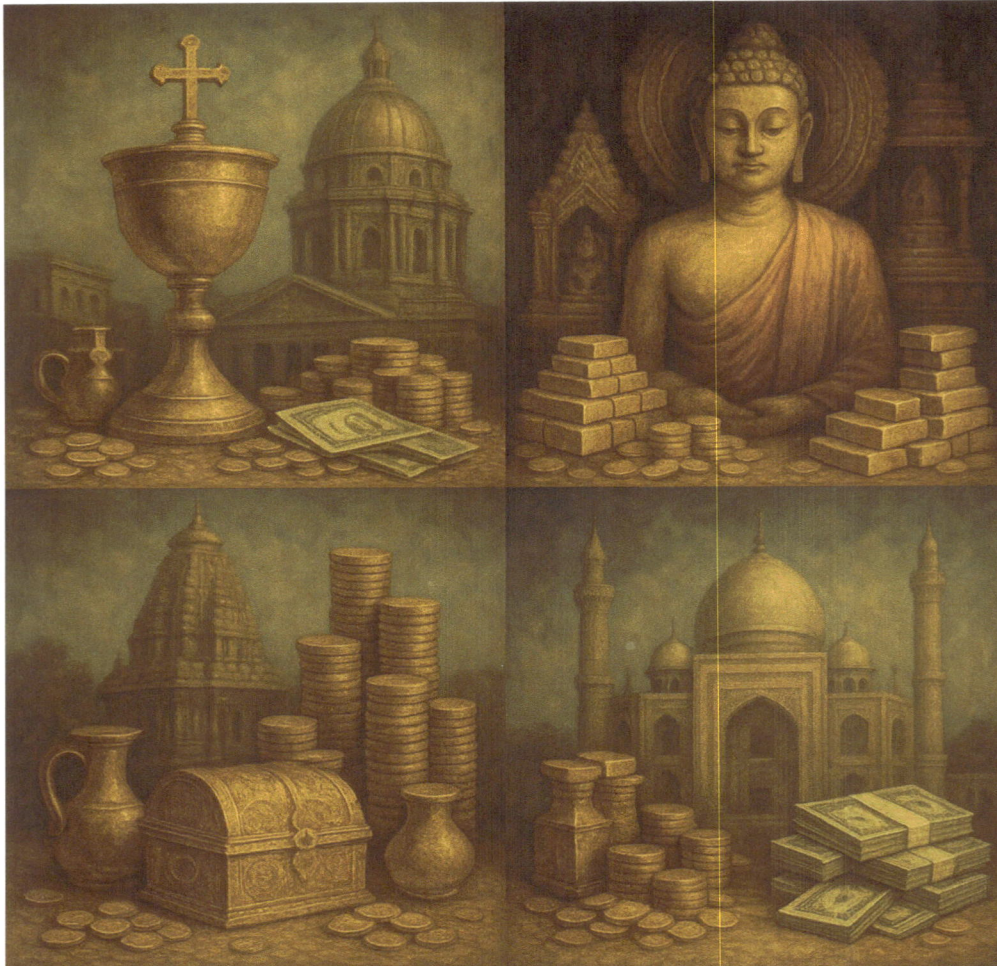

Why Does This Happen?

From a psychological and sociological standpoint, this paradox might stem from natural human tendencies:

- **Desire for Security**: Spiritual communities often accumulate resources to protect their teachings and communities from external threats.

- **Institutionalization**: Movements grow into organizations, and organizations seek stability, leading to bureaucracy and hierarchy.

- **Human Ego**: Even with the best intentions, individuals and groups may seek recognition, authority, and influence, contradicting the original teachings.

As the Tao Te Ching observes, *"The higher the structure, the farther from the Way"* (Laozi, trans. Mitchell, 1988).

Cultural Relevance Today

Today's society, riddled with consumerism, curated self-images, and institutional distrust, mirrors these spiritual paradoxes. Many seekers are disillusioned with religious structures not because they reject faith, but because they crave *authenticity*.

Holistic health practitioners recognize that wellness is found in true balance of mind, body, and spirit, and requires stripping away external noise and realigning with essential truths. It's not in grandeur but in simplicity that healing often occurs.

The example of figures like Jesus, Buddha, and Muhammad calls us back not to ritualized identity, but to the living essence of humility, compassion, and conscious living.

A Personal Reflection

This reflection isn't a condemnation of all spiritual institutions. Rather, it is a call to vigilance:

- Are we aligning with the heart of spiritual wisdom or merely its outer forms?
- Are we living simply, authentically, and compassionately, or becoming entangled in ego, status, and recognition?

As individuals seeking holistic well-being, we are invited to live in *the spirit* rather than merely follow *the form*.

Spiritual maturity requires discernment and choosing the inward journey over external display, whether in religion, health, or daily life.

References:

Esposito, J. L. (1998). *Islam: The straight path* (3rd ed.). Oxford University Press.
Flood, G. (1996). *An introduction to Hinduism*. Cambridge University Press.
Lopez, D. S., Jr. (2001). *THE STORY OF BUDDHISM*. HarperSanFrancisco.
http://www.chanreads.org/wp-content/uploads/2022/09/The-Story-of-Buddhism-A-Concise-Guide-to-Its-History-Teachings-Donald-S.-Lopez-Jr.-chanreads.org_.pdf

MacCulloch, D. (2011). *Christianity: The first three thousand years*. Penguin Books.

Mitchell, S. (Trans.). (1988). *Tao Te Ching* (Lao Tzu). Harper & Row.
The Holy Bible, New International Version. (2011). Biblica, Inc. (Original work published 1978)

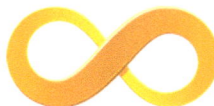

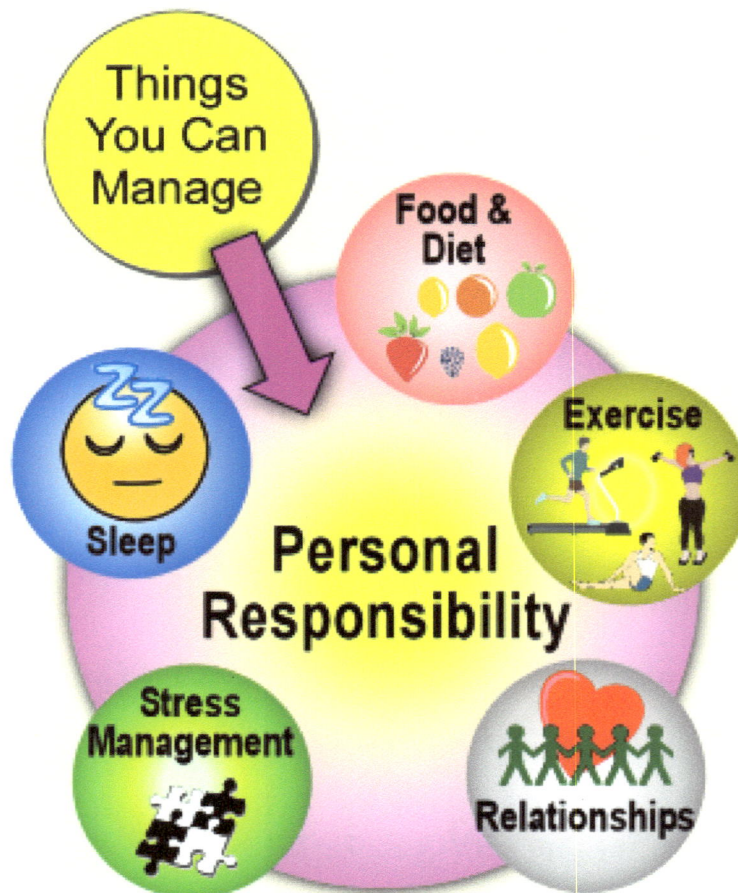

Highest Preventable Risk Factors

1) Poor diet
2) Inactivity
3) Smoking

Things You Can Manage

Food & Diet

Exercise

Sleep

Personal Responsibility

Stress Management

Relationships

www.MindAndBodyExercises.com

"Follow the science"…..maybe also "follow the data".

Move beyond thinking that your health and well-being are someone else's responsibility. Be more active, eat healthier, sleep better, stress less – these are the key components to maintaining a strong immune system.

Is Returning to "Normal" Really a Good Thing?

"Normal" in the US

- 12.2% of adults meet the daily fruit intake recommendation (CDC 2018)
- 9.3% of adults meet the daily vegetable intake recommendation (CDC 2018)
- 23% Exercise regularly (CDC 2018)
- 42% vitamin D deficiency (CDC 2018)
- 73% overweight (CDC 2018)
- 42% obese (CDC 2018)
- 18% obesity age 2-18 (CDC 2018)
- 70% on prescriptions (CDC 2019)
- 60% have chronic issues (CDC 2019)
- 40% have more than one chronic issues (comorbidities) (CDC 2019)
- 14% Smoke (CDC 2019)

Leading Causes of Death
(most preventable through lifestyle)

1) Heart disease: 690,882
2) Cancer: 598,932
3) Medical errors: 250,000-444,000 (John Hopkins 2016)
3) COVID-19: 345,323
3) Accidents (unintentional injuries): 192,176
4) Chronic lower respiratory diseases: 151,637
5) Stroke (cerebrovascular diseases): 159,050
6) Alzheimer's disease: 133,382
7) Diabetes: 101,106
8) Kidney diseased: 52,260
9) Influenza and pneumonia: 53,495
10) Intentional self-harm (suicide): 44,834
Source: CDC 2020

Highest Preventable Risk Factors

1) Poor diet
2) Inactivity
3) Smoking

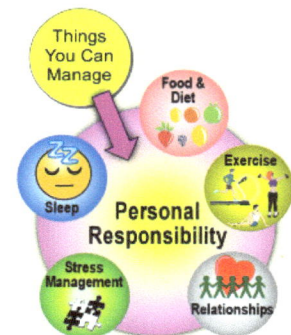

Chronic Diseases: Often Preventable, Frequently Manageable Many chronic diseases could be prevented, delayed, or alleviated, through simple lifestyle changes. The U.S. Centers for Disease Control and Prevention (CDC) estimates that eliminating three risk factors – poor diet, inactivity, and smoking – would prevent: 80% of heart disease and stroke; 80% of type 2 diabetes; and, 40% of cancer.

Obesity steals more years than diabetes, tobacco, high blood pressure and high cholesterol -- the other top preventable health problems that cut Americans' lives short, according to researchers who analyzed 2014 data.

If not being sick is the goal, we need to focus on being fit, well & healthy

www.MindAndBodyExercises.com

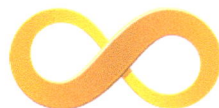

Iatrogenesis – 3rd Leading Cause of Death in US

Meriam-Webster defines iatrogenesis as "inadvertent and preventable induction of disease or complications by the medical treatment or procedures of a physician or surgeon" (Iatrogenesis, n.d.)

Number of Deaths in the United States

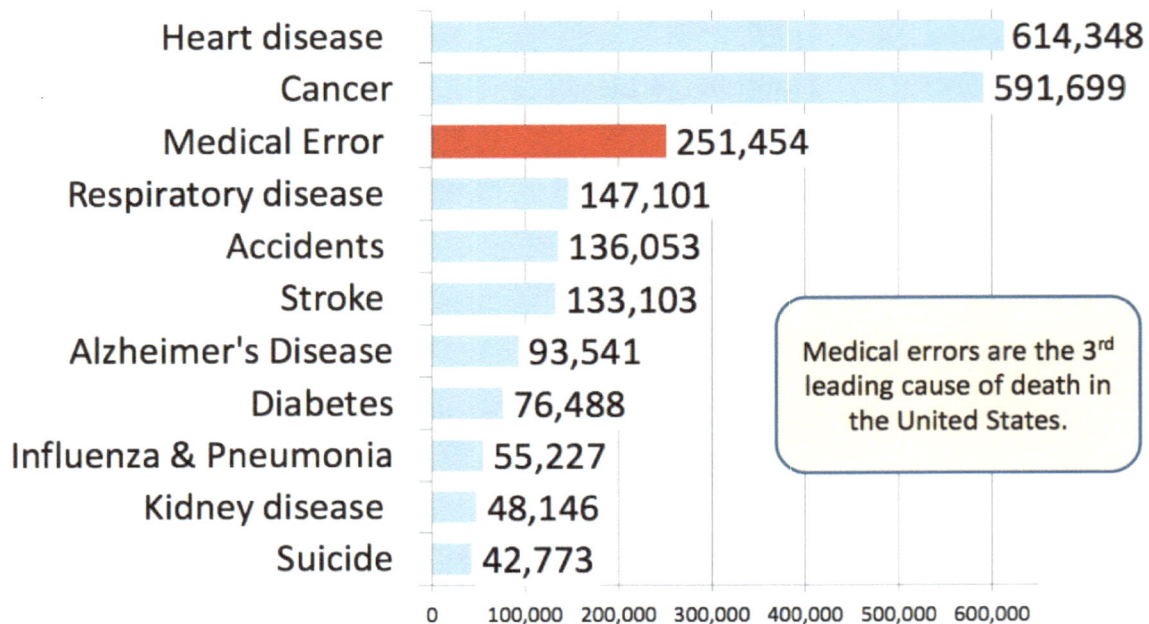

Cause	Deaths
Heart disease	614,348
Cancer	591,699
Medical Error	251,454
Respiratory disease	147,101
Accidents	136,053
Stroke	133,103
Alzheimer's Disease	93,541
Diabetes	76,488
Influenza & Pneumonia	55,227
Kidney disease	48,146
Suicide	42,773

Medical errors are the 3rd leading cause of death in the United States.

Sources: CDC. National Center for Health Statistics. Number of deaths for leading causes of death, 2014.

The following excerpt is from Marc Micozzi's Fundamentals of Complementary, Alternative, and Integrative Medicine:

In 1847, partially in response to the acceptance and success of homeopathy, and after prior attempts, a group of regular physicians founded an organization to serve as the unifying body for orthodox medical practitioners. The American Medical Association (AMA), initially under Nathaniel Chapman, was founded in Philadelphia. Physicians who belonged to the AMA considered themselves regular practitioners and adhered to therapeutics termed heroic medicine (Rutkow and Rutkow, 2004). Their invasive treatments distinguished these regular doctors to their patients. They often consisted of bleeding and blistering in addition to administering harsh concoctions to induce vomiting and purging. These treatments at the time were considered state of the art.

The justification behind such harsh treatments was a commitment to a scientific materialist medical theory, actually moving away from empirically based, "rational" medicine. Regular doctors did not share belief in the concept of the healing power of nature (the vis medicatrix naturae), and felt that a physician's duty was to provide active, "heroic" intervention. Despite this attitude, patients recovered notwithstanding their treatments. This reality had the ironic effect of encouraging both regular doctors' belief in heroic treatments and natural doctors' belief in the inborn capacity for self-healing, despite the further injuries caused by many regular treatments. Much like physicians today are pressured to provide an active treatment that may sometimes be unnecessary (such as prescribing an antibiotic for a viral infection), regular doctors of the 1800s also felt pressure to give the heroic treatments for which they were known. James Whorton (2002) wrotes, "it was only natural for MDs to close ranks and cling more tightly to that tradition as a badge of professional identity, making depletive therapy the core of their self-image as medical orthodoxy."

Although the AMA initially held no legal authority (like the multiplying medical subspecialty practice associations of today), it began a major push during the second half of the nineteenth century to create legislation and standards of medical education and competency. This process culminated in 1910 with the publication of Medical Education in the United States and Canada, compiled by Abraham Flexner (Fig. 21.2), also known as the Flexner Report. It has been described as "a bombshell that rattled medical and political forces throughout the country" (Petrina, 2008). It criticized the medical education of its era as a loose and poorly structured apprenticeship system that generally lacked any defined standards or goals beyond commercialism (Ober, 1997). In some of his specific accounts, Flexner described medical institutions as "utterly wretched … without a redeeming feature" and as "a hopeless affair" (Whorton, 2002). Many regular medical institutions were rated poorly, and most of the irregular "alternative" schools fared the worst. After this report, nearly half of the medical schools in the country closed, and by 1930 the remaining schools had 4-year programs of rigorous "scientific medicine."

Following the Flexner Report, a tremendous restructuring of medical education and practice occurred. The remaining medical schools experienced enormous growth: in 1910 a leading school might have had a budget of $ 100,000; by 1965 it was $ 20 million, and by 1990 it would have been $ 200 million or more (Ludmerer, 1999). Faculty were now called on to engage in original research, and students not only studied a curriculum with a heavy emphasis on science, but also engaged in active learning by participating in real clinical work with responsibility for patients. Hospitals became the locus for clinical instruction. As scientific discovery began to accelerate, these higher educational standards helped to bridge the gap between what was known and what was put into practice. More stringent licensing and independent testing provided a greater degree of confidence in the competence of the nation's doctors. During this same time period, the suppression and decline of alternative schools of health care occurred, as both public and political pressure increased.

The 1910 Flexner Report, sponsored by the Carnegie Foundation, compared all American medical schools against a standard represented by the new Johns Hopkins University School of Medicine, which had been founded in 1888. Criticism was so devastating that about three-quarters of American medical schools closed, including many osteopathic medical schools.

Bernarr Macfadden, founded the "physical culture" school of health and healing, also known as physcultopathy. This school of healing gave birth across the United States to gymnasiums where exercise programs were designed and taught to allow individual men and women to establish and maintain optimal physical health.

Although so strongly based on common sense and observation, many theories exist to explain the rapid dissolution of these diverse healing arts. The practitioners at one time made up more than 25% of all U.S. health care practitioners in the early part of the twentieth century. Low ratings in the infamous Flexner Report (which ranked all these schools of medical thought among the lowest), allopathic medicine's anointing of itself with the blessing "scientific," and the growing political sophistication of the AMA clearly played significant roles. Of course, the acceptance of the germ theory of disease and development of effective antibiotics for the first time provided a strong rationale for the new, "scientific," regular medicine.

> Let's face it, in America today we don't have a health care system, we have a sick care system. We wait until people become obese, develop chronic diseases, or become disabled – and then we spend untold hundreds of billions annually to try to make them better.
>
> Tom Harkin

Additionally:

Whatever the validity of medical critiques, the American medical establishment's policy on chiropractic was not that of a disinterested group seeking to serve the public health and well-being. A century-long campaign against chiropractic impeded medical advancement and at times posed a severe threat. Until relatively recently, allopathic medical students were taught that chiropractic is harmful, or at best worthless, and they in turn passed along these prejudices to their own patients.

A staunchly anti-chiropractic policy was pursued by the American Medical Association (AMA). In 1990 the U.S. Supreme Court affirmed a lower court ruling in which the AMA was found liable for federal antitrust violations for having engaged in a conspiracy to "contain and eliminate" (the AMA's own words) the chiropractic profession (Wilk v. AMA, 1990). The process that culminated in this landmark decision began in 1974 when a large packet of confidential AMA documents was provided anonymously to leaders of the American Chiropractic Association and the International Chiropractors Association. As a result of the ensuing Wilk v. AMA litigation, the AMA reversed its long-standing ban on interprofessional cooperation between medical doctors and chiropractors, agreed to publish the full findings of the court in the Journal of the American Medical Association, and paid an undisclosed sum, most of which was earmarked for chiropractic research. This ruling has not completely reversed the effects of organized medicine's boycott, especially when it comes to the application of the most effective and cost-effective treatments for common pain conditions.

There is good and bad in all things, depending upon the circumstances for whatever situation presents itself. If an arm is severed, a bone is crushed or traumatic injuries – get immediate medical help. If you suffer from allergies, back pain, headaches and a plethora of other non-life-threatening issues – become educated as to what options are available. Be well, become healthy, be wise.

References:

Anderson, J. G., & Abrahamson, K. (2017). Your Health Care May Kill You: Medical Errors. Studies in health technology and informatics, 234, 13–17.
iatrogenesis. (n.d.). The Merriam-Webster.Com Dictionary. Retrieved August 17, 2022, from https://www.merriam-webster.com/medical/iatrogenesis

Micozzi, Marc S.. Fundamentals of Complementary, Alternative, and Integrative Medicine – E-Book (p. 537). Elsevier Health Sciences. Kindle Edition.

Micozzi, Marc S.. Fundamentals of Complementary, Alternative, and Integrative Medicine – E-Book (p. 644). Elsevier Health Sciences. Kindle Edition.

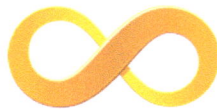

10-90% of the Efficacy of Prescriptions Comes Down to the Placebo Effect

Our society seems to rely heavily upon interpretation of scientific data, when it comes to healthcare and guidance, relative pharmaceuticals, procedures, etc. However, it is ironic that the US healthcare system relies quite heavily on this perception that medical pharmaceuticals can fix many ailments. The power of suggestion can play a significant role in alleviating pain and suffering. Somewhere between 10-90% of the efficacy of prescriptions comes down to the placebo effect.

Factors such as trust in the doctor prescribing the medication, specific details regarding the medicine, like its brand, price, name, and place of origin can all affect the patient's potential belief in the medicine improving their aliment. So, while we keep hearing "follow the science", the science seems to show that the placebo effect is indeed real and part of the US healthcare system.

External context

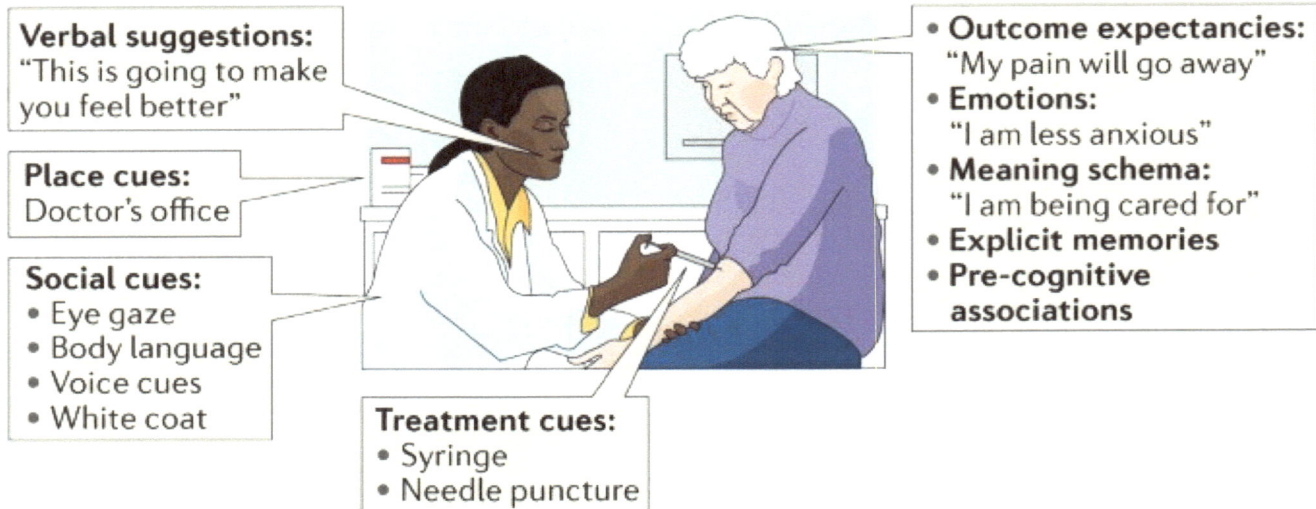

Verbal suggestions:
"This is going to make you feel better"

Place cues:
Doctor's office

Social cues:
• Eye gaze
• Body language
• Voice cues
• White coat

Treatment cues:
• Syringe
• Needle puncture

Internal context

• **Outcome expectancies:**
"My pain will go away"
• **Emotions:**
"I am less anxious"
• **Meaning schema:**
"I am being cared for"
• **Explicit memories**
• **Pre-cognitive associations**

Nature Reviews | Neuroscience

References:

Colloca L. (2019). The Placebo Effect in Pain Therapies. Annual review of pharmacology and toxicology, 59, 191–211. https://doi.org/10.1146/annurev-pharmtox-010818-021542

The Pharmaceutical Journal, PJ, 19 September 2015, Vol 295, No 7880;295(7880):DOI:10.1211/PJ.2015.20069282
https://www.nature.com/articles/nrn3976

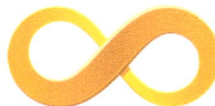

The 3 Healthcare Systems in the US

1 – "Health-care" which is truly "sick-care"

2 – "Self-care"

3 – "I Don't Care"

Be more active, eat healthier, sleep better, stress less these are the key components to maintaining a strong immune system.

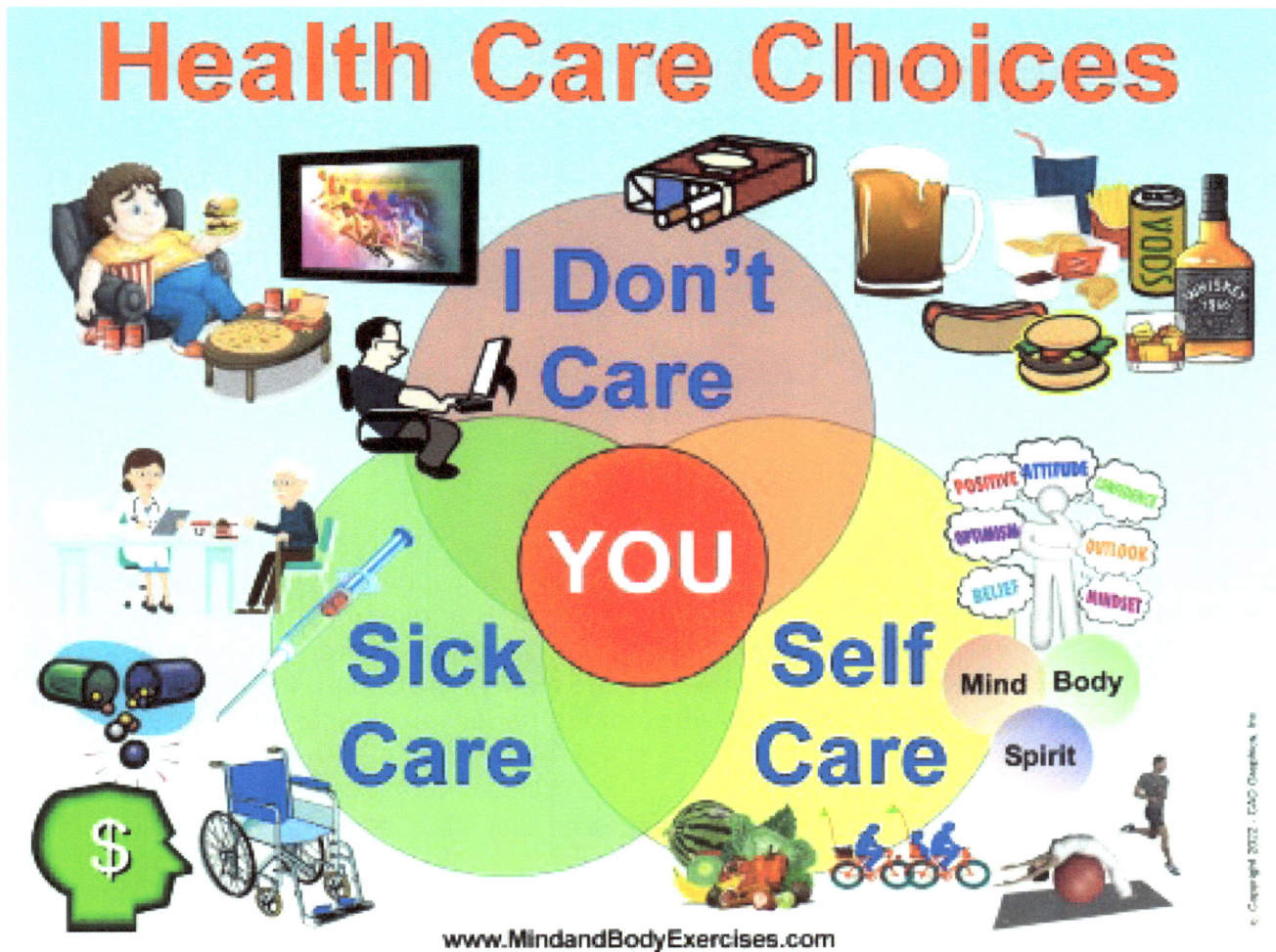

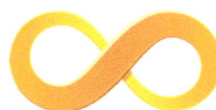

www.MindandBodyExercises.com

In the age of evidence-based medicine, published research is often viewed as the gold standard for guiding health decisions. However, behind the polished language of medical journals lies a complex web of funding, publication bias, and editorial politics. While many researchers uphold high standards, recent investigations reveal systemic vulnerabilities in how medical studies are published, even in the world's most respected journals.

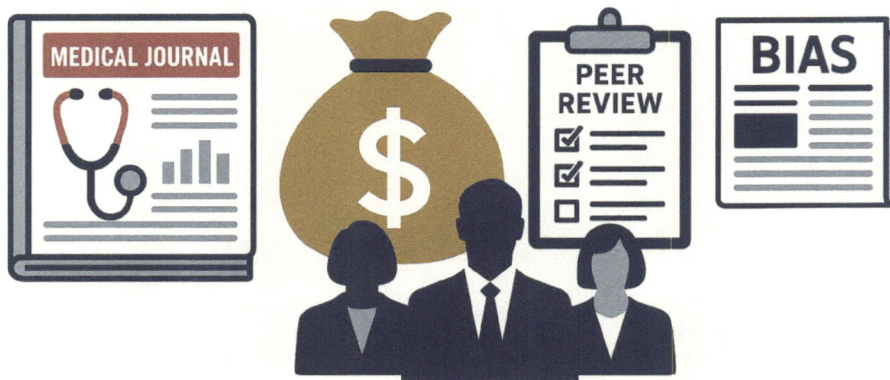

The Traditional Path to Publication

Medical studies generally follow a structured path to publication. Researchers begin by designing their study, obtaining ethical approval (e.g., IRB approval), and collecting data. A manuscript is then submitted to a peer-reviewed journal, where it undergoes scrutiny by field experts who evaluate its methodology, novelty, and clarity. The editorial team, taking reviewer feedback into account, decides whether the paper will be accepted, revised, or rejected.

This peer-review process is intended to serve as a quality filter. However, peer reviewers are unpaid, overburdened, and not always able to detect fraudulent or misleading work, especially in fields outside their specialty (Smith, 2006).

The Cost of Getting Published

One of the less visible aspects of medical publishing is the cost. While traditional journals may publish accepted articles without charge, many newer or open-access journals charge "article processing charges" (APCs) that range from $1,500 to over $5,000 per article (Solomon & Björk, 2012). These fees are often covered by research grants or institutional funding, but they can also create barriers for independent researchers and incentivize some journals to accept more articles, compromising rigor for revenue.

Moreover, the push toward open-access publishing has led to the rise of predatory journals, where publications charge authors but lack credible peer review. This has flooded the academic ecosystem with poorly vetted studies that masquerade as legitimate science.

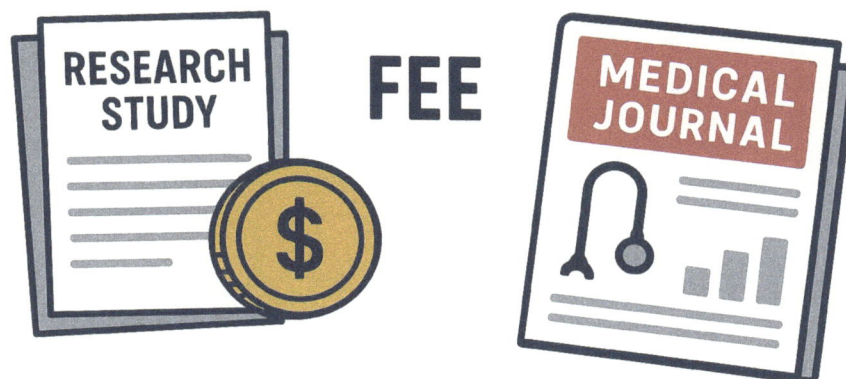

Politics and Prestige in Editorial Decisions

Studies have shown that research from prestigious universities is more likely to be accepted for publication, a phenomenon known as the "Matthew Effect" (Merton, 1968). Additionally, journals tend to favor studies with statistically significant or "positive" results, leading to a well-documented "publication bias" (Dwan et al., 2013). Negative findings, though scientifically valuable, are less likely to be published, skewing the evidence base.
Even more concerning, high-impact journals have been shown to favor topics that align with social trends or commercial interests. For instance, an investigation by *The Wall Street Journal* in 2005 exposed how pharmaceutical companies employed ghostwriters to author studies that promoted their drugs, later assigning authorship to respected academics to add legitimacy (Armstrong, 2005). This practice, while not universally accepted, was alarmingly common at the time.

The Paper Mill Problem

In 2024, *The Wall Street Journal* released another bombshell: a flood of fraudulent research papers had forced the publisher Wiley to retract over 11,000 articles and shut down 19 academic journals (Marcus & Overland, 2024). These papers were often generated by "paper mills" which are organizations that produce fake scientific studies for a fee. Some even used AI to generate content that mimicked legitimate science, exposing deep vulnerabilities in the peer-review and editorial process.

This was not an isolated incident. Other publishers, including Elsevier and Taylor & Francis, have faced similar challenges, revealing how even major journals can be infiltrated by illegitimate science when editorial oversight fails.

The Problem with "Trust the Science"

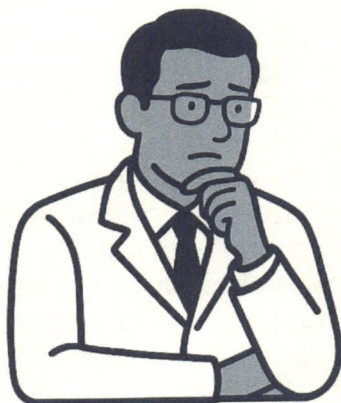

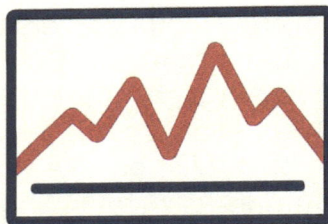

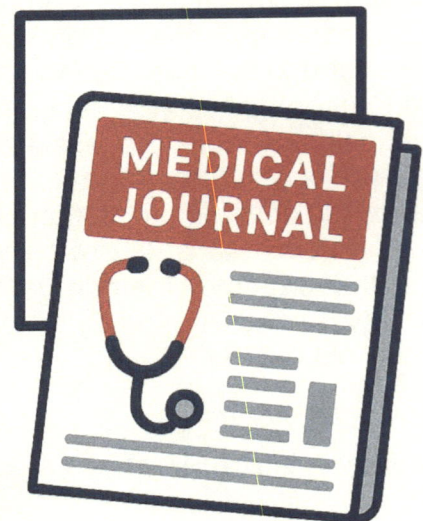

In recent years, the phrase **"trust the science"** has become a cultural catchphrase used by media, governments, and institutions to affirm confidence in scientific guidance. While well-intentioned, this phrase can be misleading. It implies that science is monolithic and settled, when in fact it is a dynamic process subject to debate, revision, and crucially, accessibility. Not all valid scientific perspectives make it to publication. Financial constraints, editorial preferences, and publication bias mean that some high-quality studies are never seen by the public or professionals. This selective visibility creates an illusion of consensus, when in reality many opposing findings may have been filtered out of the mainstream conversation (Dwan et al., 2013). Thus, trusting "the science" too literally can obscure the fact that what gets published is only a portion of what is known or could be known on any given topic.

TRUST THE SCIENCE?

POLITICS AND PEER REVIEW

SUBSTANTIAL PUBLICATION FEES

SELECTIVE REPORTING

MEDICAL JOURNAL

A Historical Case: Vioxx and the NEJM

Concerns over editorial bias are not new. In 2006, *The Wall Street Journal* reported on how the *New England Journal of Medicine* failed to detect misleading data about the arthritis drug Vioxx, which was later withdrawn from the market due to cardiovascular risks (Martinez & Winslow, 2006). Critics argued that key risk data were omitted from published studies, undermining public safety.

This case became a turning point in the debate over transparency, conflict of interest, and pharmaceutical influence in academic publishing.

Navigating the Landscape: A Call for Awareness

For health-conscious individuals and practitioners in holistic wellness, the takeaway is not to reject scientific research, but to read it critically. The peer-reviewed system has value, but it is not infallible. Consider the funding source, author affiliations, and whether the journal itself is reputable and transparent about its processes.

Advocates for scientific reform are pushing for stronger peer-review standards, post-publication review systems, and the full disclosure of data and conflicts of interest. Platforms like *Retraction Watch*, *PubPeer*, and preprint servers like *medRxiv* offer tools for transparency.

- Retraction Watch
- PubPeer
- MedRxiv
- PLOS ONE Publication Criteria
- WSJ science reporting

References:

Armstrong, D. (2005, December 13). At medical journals, writers paid by industry play big role. *The Wall Street Journal*. https://www.wsj.com/articles/SB113443606745420770

Dwan, K., Gamble, C., Williamson, P. R., & Kirkham, J. J. (2013). Systematic review of the empirical evidence of study publication bias and outcome reporting bias—An updated review. *PLOS ONE, 8*(7), e66844. https://doi.org/10.1371/journal.pone.0066844

Marcus, A., & Overland, C. (2024, February 22). Flood of fake science forces multiple journal closures. *The Wall Street Journal*. https://www.wsj.com/science/academic-studies-research-paper-mills-journals-publishing-f5a3d4bc

Martinez, B., & Winslow, R. (2006, May 18). How the New England Journal missed warning signs on Vioxx. *The Wall Street Journal*. https://www.wsj.com/articles/SB114765430315252591

Merton, R. K. (1968). The Matthew effect in science: The reward and communication systems of science are considered. *Science, 159*(3810), 56–63. https://doi.org/10.1126/science.159.3810.56

Smith, R. (2006). Peer review: A flawed process at the heart of science and journals. *Journal of the Royal Society of Medicine, 99*(4), 178–182. https://doi.org/10.1258/jrsm.99.4.178

Solomon, D. J., & Björk, B. C. (2012). A study of open access journals using article processing charges. *Journal of the American Society for Information Science and Technology, 63*(8), 1485–1495. https://doi.org/10.1002/asi.22673

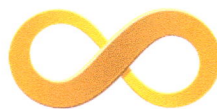

have commented on this topic in former discussions, specifically big pharmaceutical companies hindering expansion of the herbal market, where they either buy out the smaller herbal companies or use their vast resources to lobby against or stifle growth of alternative natural medicinal options. I really don't think it is wise to take a 'let's wait and see where this goes" approach as opposed to a "be self-reliant in pursuing natural options through due diligence" type of attitude. I feel people need to be more accountable to themselves and their loved ones, for managing their own healthcare or more appropriately "self-care" program. Herbs and other natural remedies will continue to see more re-acceptance and growth as people increasingly become weary of the high costs, side-effects and politics associated with pharmaceuticals. This is evident from a past article on the global herbal medicine market is predicted to possibly become a $550 billion industry by 2030 (insightSLICE, 2021).

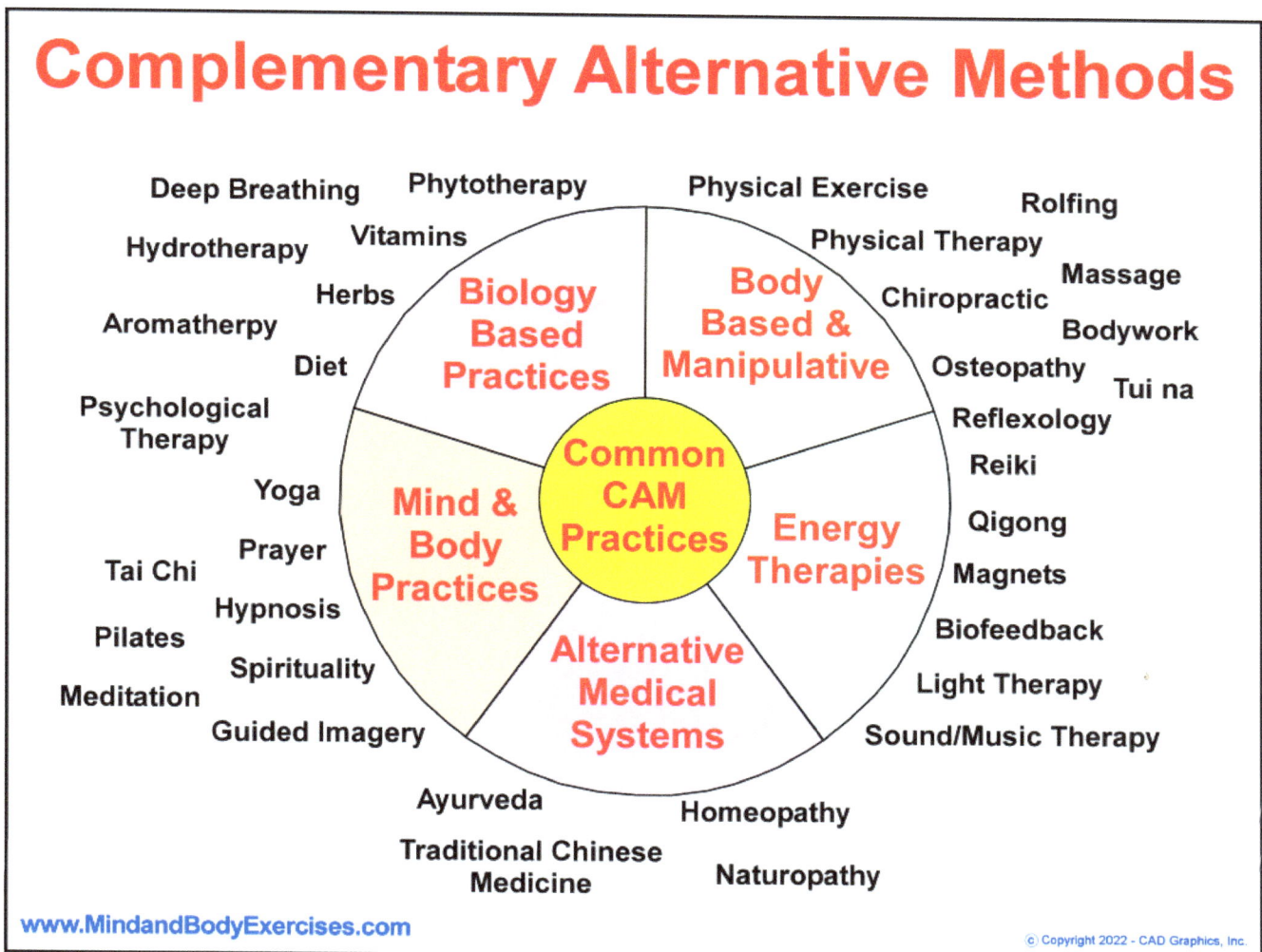

www.MindandBodyExercises.com

© Copyright 2022 - CAD Graphics, Inc.

From my own experience, Western medical professionals are not going to offer or steer a patient towards herbs when the whole healthcare industry is based upon mostly quick-fix pharmaceuticals and most often at exorbitantly higher costs to the consumer. For example, my allopathic doctor prescribed Nasacort, Flonase and eventually Claritin for seasonal allergies, when I was able to replace these with a combination of ginger, turmeric and black pepper with great success. Another orthopedic doctor was intent upon me having surgery for a torn meniscus in my knee. I declined and practiced more qigong and applied herbs topically to my injured knee for 6 months, again with much success.

My botanical medicine history started when my mother gave me warm milk with honey for a sore throat when I was probably 4 or 5 years old. My mother's family came from what was formerly known as Bohemia and now named the Czech Republic, and my father's ancestors came from Germany, where decades back traditional medicines and herbal remedies were quite common. Around this same time, I was introduced to Jägermeister (probably considered child abuse these days), the alcoholic beverage that actually has medicinal properties from its herbal ingredients of cinnamon, ginger root, licorice root and rose hips (Arifin, 2017).

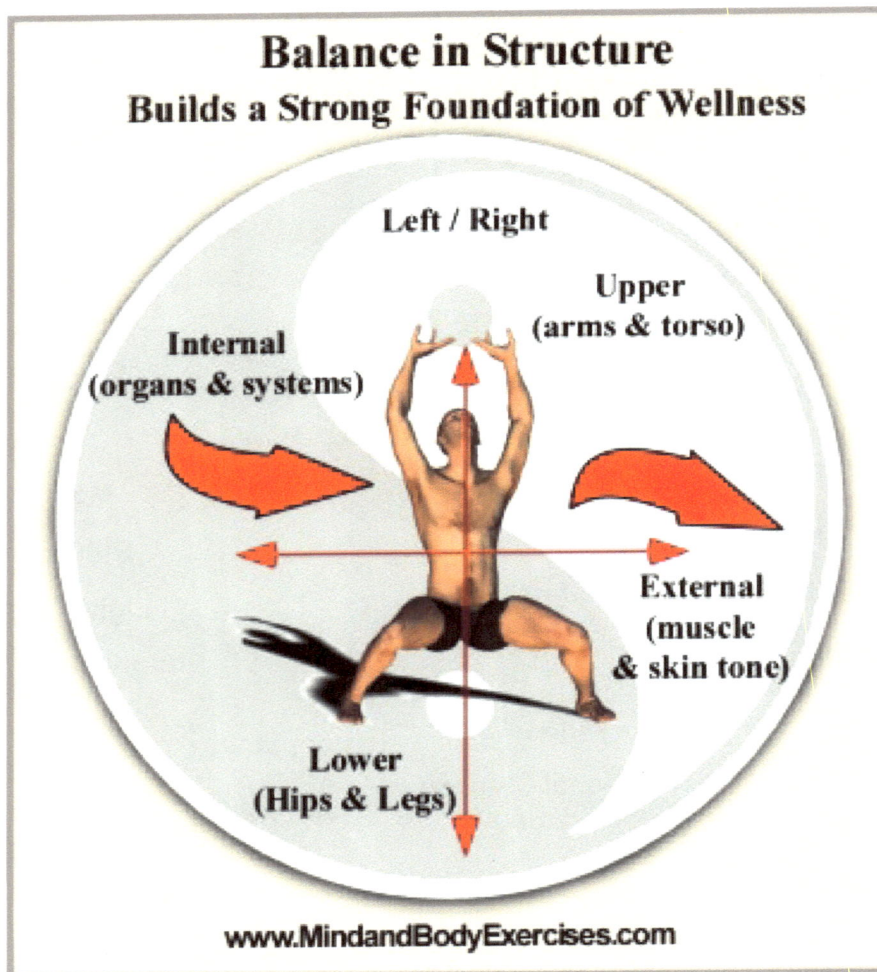

Balance in Structure
Builds a Strong Foundation of Wellness

Left / Right

Upper (arms & torso)

Internal (organs & systems)

External (muscle & skin tone)

Lower (Hips & Legs)

www.MindandBodyExercises.com

Years later when I was 16, I began martial arts training with Korean and Chinese kung fu. My teachers were very much Taoists and Traditional Chinese Medicine was inherently bound within our curriculum and knowledge base. I was quite naïve and impressionable at the time, having had little true-life experience. Fortunately for me, this was a very good education to have been introduced to at such an early age, as it gave me a firm foundation in health, fitness, wellness and nutrition for years to come.

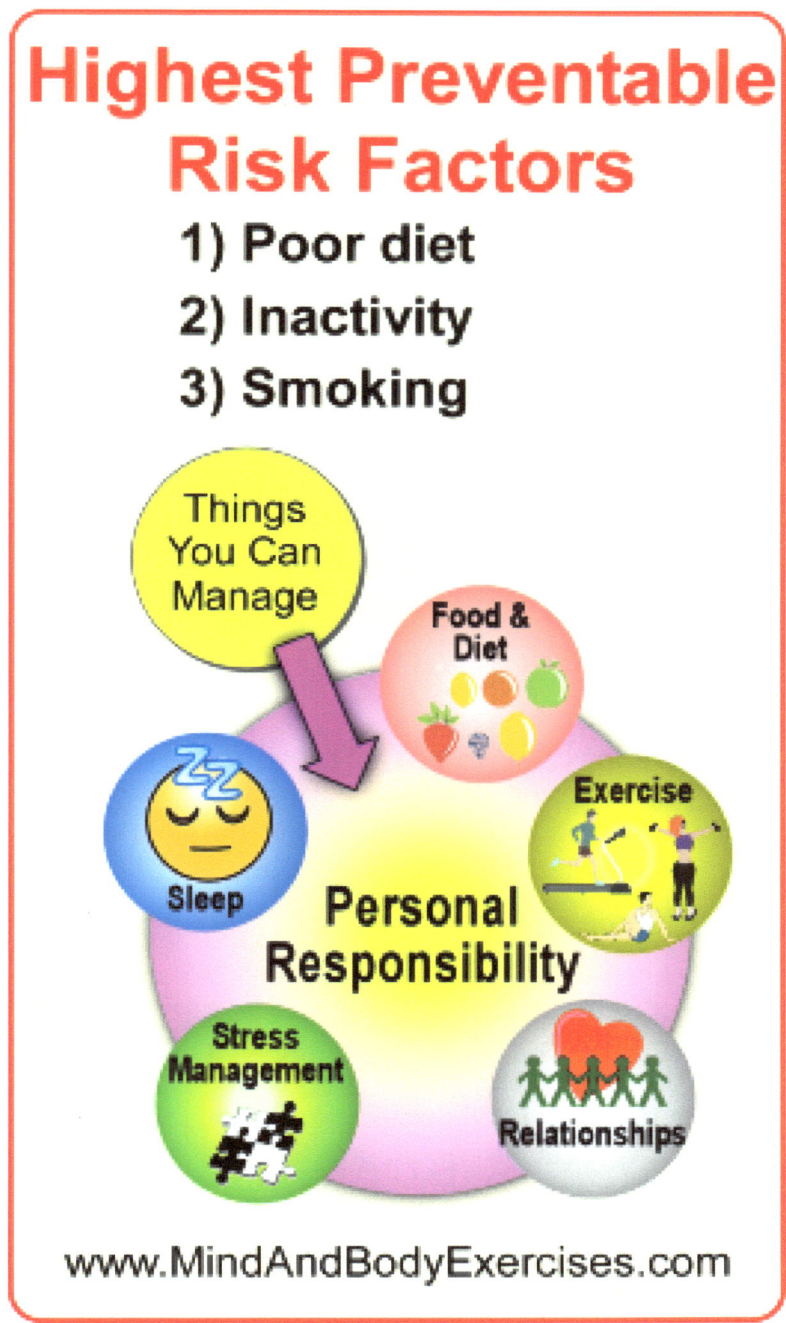

Highest Preventable Risk Factors

1) Poor diet
2) Inactivity
3) Smoking

Things You Can Manage

Food & Diet

Exercise

Sleep

Personal Responsibility

Stress Management

Relationships

www.MindAndBodyExercises.com

I was taught (along with my peers and fellow students) that the body can innately maintain and cure itself if given the right balance of physical exercise, proper diet and nutrition (including herbs) and appropriate self-management of our thoughts and emotions. Our go to beverage and preventative, was ginger root tea, to aid in good digestion and overall reduction of inflammation relative to physical training. If overly sore or injured, we would use curcumin poultices or store-bought plaster patches with cayenne. We would use herbal extracts called Dit Da Jow, to apply to our hands, arms and other parts of our bodies for what is referred to as Iron Body training. These Jows are somewhat unique in that they reduce inflammation while at the same time increase blood circulation and promote natural healing. We ate kimchi, a known probiotic and were encouraged to eat and cook with garlic, ginger, turmeric, cayenne and onion as much as possible.

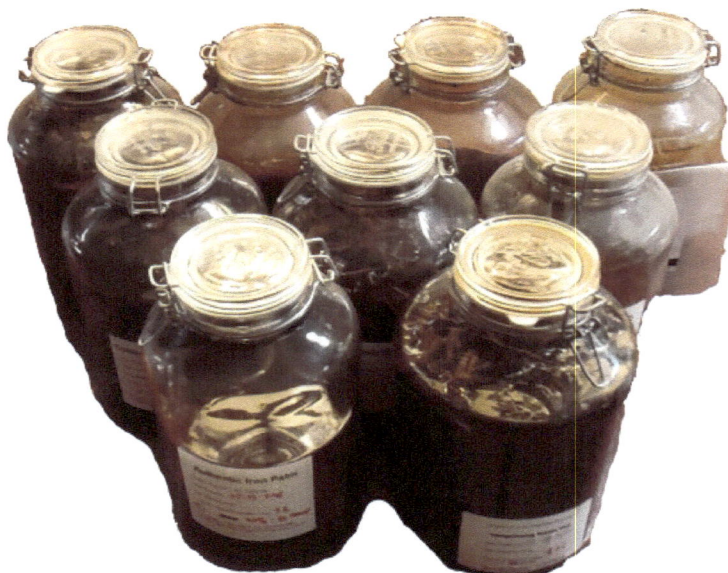

Years later, the training and knowledge increased to even more Traditional Chinese Medicine methods of moxibustion. This is a method, where herbs smolder on acupuncture needles or sometimes directly on the skin (direct moxibustion) or indirect where the herbs burn on a layer of ginger, garlic or salt which cover specific acupuncture points and meridians.

Additionally, we were prescribed or instructed on how to use particular Chinese herbal tea recipes for various physical imbalances. These teas were incredibly strong in flavor and potency, and were to help cure whatever issues of cough, allergies, tinnitus, irritable bowel syndrome, headache, and many other ailments. These teas looked like tar by the time they decocted down to a cup size serving and tasted pretty much the same, but they all worked amazingly well. Even more recently, I have been introduced to Ayurveda through my martial arts lineage as well as with my NVU degree program. Ayurveda seems to be the parent of TCM in many aspects, as I have found many of the same herbs and principles of treatment and prevention from using specific recipes.

I have been fully into the whole concept of phytotherapy for almost 50 years, for all of the reasons I have discussed over previous posts, distilling it down to less side effects, less toxins, less cost, more individual control over my own health and well-being. I see herbalism/botanical addressing the root causes of illness and disease as well as symptoms, versus conventional allopathic medicine treating the symptoms with little or no expectation of addressing root issues. Herbalism seems to have its greatest benefits as a preventative for chronic and long-term ailments, however having benefits for some acute issues also. Conventional allopathic medicine's greatest strength is in immediate treatment for trauma and acute illnesses.

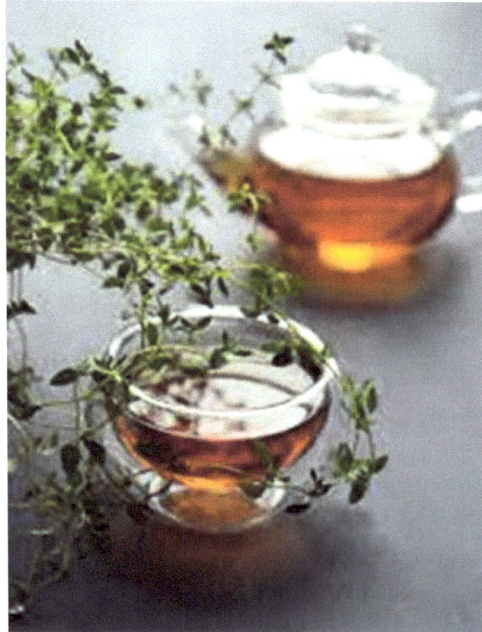

References:

Arifin, E. (2017, December 23). 7 Health Benefits of Drinking Jagermeister #1 Unexpected. DrHealthBenefits.com. https://drhealthbenefits.com/food-bevarages/beverages/health-benefits-drinking-jagermeister

insightSLICE. (2021, February 16). Herbal Medicine Market Global Sales Are Expected To Reach US$ 550 Billion by 2030, as stated by insightSLICE. GlobeNewswire News Room. https://www.globenewswire.com/news-release/2021/02/16/2176036/0/en/Herbal-Medicine-Market-Global-Sales-Are-Expected-To-Reach-US-550-Billion-by-2030-as-stated-by-insightSLICE.html

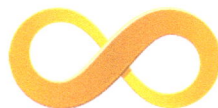

SECTION II: EASTERN & HOLISTIC PHILOSOPHY

Understanding the Evolution of Supreme Principles in Daoist Cosmology

In the study of Daoist philosophy and traditional Chinese thought, the term "Tai Chi" (太極) is widely recognized as referring to the **Supreme Ultimate**, a foundational principle in the universe from which all dualities (*yin* and *yang*) arise (Liao,1990).

Practitioners of Tai Chi Chuan may know the term as associated with martial arts, yet its roots are far deeper, embedded in cosmology, metaphysics, and classical Daoist thought. But what if we go one step earlier, or even further back? What came before Tai Chi? And what of other similarly constructed terms such as *"Tai Su"* (太素) and *"Tai Yu"* (太宇)? Are they simply linguistic variants, or do they represent unique philosophical concepts in the evolution of universal principles?

Wuji (無極): The Limitless Void

In the beginning was **Wuji**, often translated as "non-ultimate" or "limitless." Wuji represents pure potential being formless, timeless, and undivided. It is the **Dao** before manifestation (Robinet, 1997). In diagrams, Wuji is usually shown as an empty circle or a vast blank space, signifying the absence of polarity.

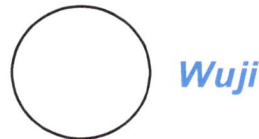

Wuji

Tai Su (太素): The Supreme Simplicity

Emerging from Wuji is **Tai Su**, a term less commonly discussed but highly significant in classical Daoist texts.

- **Tai (太)** = supreme or great

- **Su (素)** = simple, elemental, unadorned, or fundamental substance

Tai Su is understood as the primordial essence or supreme simplicity. A state where differentiation is beginning to arise but not yet fully formed. It is the first stirring of substance, the bridge between the void and duality. In *Huainanzi*, Tai Su is mentioned as a precursor to cosmic formation (Le Blanc & Mathieu, 2008). In early Chinese alchemy and cosmology, it represents the primordial *qi* that has yet to divide into yin and yang (Pregadio, 2008).

Simplicity

Tai Chi (太極): The Supreme Ultimate

When differentiation occurs, **Tai Chi** comes into being. The term, often Romanized as **Taiji**, literally means **"Supreme Ultimate."** This is the phase where the one becomes two: yin and yang emerge as complementary polarities (Liao,1990).

Tai Chi is typically symbolized by the **Taijitu**, the black-and-white "yin-yang" symbol, expressing balance, transformation, and interdependence. In this state, movement and stillness alternate, giving rise to all forms in the universe (Kirkland, 2004).

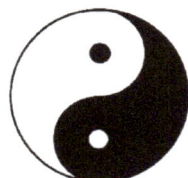

Taiiitu

Tai Yu (太宇): The Supreme Universe

Tai Yu introduces a more spatial or structural aspect to cosmology.

- **Yu (宇)** refers to the universe, cosmic space, or even the eaves of a roof, or a poetic image of a sheltering order.

- Thus, Tai Yu translates to "Supreme Universe" or "Great Cosmos."

While Tai Chi marks the origin of dynamic duality, Tai Yu is more about manifested order, and the structured universe as it exists with stars, planets, natural laws, and cycles (Graham, 1989). It is not a transitional phase but the result of the Tai Chi mechanism unfolding through space and time.

Cosmological Sequence Diagram

To visualize this progression, the accompanying diagram illustrates the unfolding of the cosmos:

1. **Wuji (無極)** – The Limitless Void

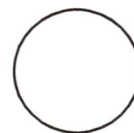

↓

2. **Tai Su (太素)** – Supreme Simplicity (undifferentiated essence)

↓

3. **Tai Chi (太極)** – Supreme Ultimate (birth of yin and yang)

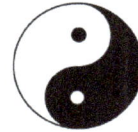

$$\downarrow$$

4. **Tai Yu (太宇)** – Supreme Universe (structured cosmos)

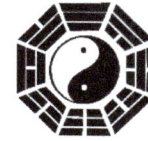

Term	Translation	Symbol	Meaning
Wuji	Limitless Void	Empty circle (○)	Undifferentiated nothingness
Tai Su	Supreme Simplicity	Solid black circle (●)	Primordial essence
Tai Chi	Supreme Ultimate	Yin-Yang (☯ / Taijitu)	Birth of duality
Tai Yu	Supreme Universe	Bagua or Heaven–Earth (八卦 / 天地)	Manifest cosmos; structured reality

Cultural and Linguistic Notes: Korean Equivalents

In Korean, these terms are written in Hanja (Chinese characters used in Korean language):

- **Tai Chi (太極)** ⟶ **Tae Guk (태극)**, as seen in the South Korean flag

- **Tai Su (太素)** ⟶ **Tae So (태소)** (rarely used in common language)

- **Tai Yu (太宇)** ⟶ **Tae U (태우)** (used in poetic or classical references)

While the philosophical usage remains mostly consistent with Chinese meanings, these terms are far less prevalent in Korean popular culture outside of Tae Guk.

Conclusion: A Philosophical Framework of Evolution

From non-being to primordial essence, and from dynamic polarity to cosmic order, this cosmological sequence illustrates how Daoist philosophy views the evolution of the universe not as a chaotic explosion, but as an elegant, cyclical, and ordered unfolding.
Whether you are a practitioner of martial arts, a student of Daoist metaphysics, or a

philosopher of natural laws, understanding Wuji ⟶ Tai Su ⟶ Tai Chi ⟶ Tai Yu offers a powerful lens through which to view the origin of all things and your own place within the ever-unfolding Tao.

Important to note, in martial arts culture, Tai chi, Tai Su, Tai Yu, Tae Guk and Tai Chi Chung are all very different forms of mental, physical and spiritual practices. While some may share some similarities, anyone who has deeply studied and practiced these methods is aware of their varying nuances and complexities.

Term	Characters	Translation	Philosophical Meaning
Wuji	無極	Non-Ultimate / Limitless	The primordial void; pure potential without polarity
Tai Su	太素	Supreme Simplicity / Primordial Essence	Undifferentiated, fundamental matter—precursor to form and duality
Tai Chi	太極	Supreme Ultimate	The origin of duality (yin and yang); dynamic balance
Tai Yu	太宇	Supreme Universe / Great Cosmos	The structured universe or cosmic order that emerges after duality

References:

Blanc, C. L., & Mathieu, R. (2008). Approches critiques de la mythologie chinoise. https://doi.org/10.4000/books.pum.19027

Graham, A. C. (1989). *Disputers of the Tao: Philosophical Argument in Ancient China*. Open Court.

Kirkland, R. (2004). *Taoism: The Enduring Tradition*. Routledge.

Pregadio, F. (2008). The Encyclopedia of Taoism. Routledge.

Robinet, I. (1997). *Taoism: Growth of a Religion*. Stanford University Press.
Liao, W. (n.d.). T'ai chi classics. Shambhala. https://www.shambhala.com/t-ai-chi-classics.html

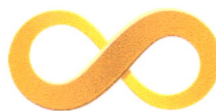

For centuries, Chinese culture has been shaped by a triad of the philosophical systems of **Confucianism**, **Taoism**, and **Buddhism**. Though distinct in their teachings, they are often seen as complementary threads that weave together a balanced and meaningful life. Each offers a unique focus: Confucianism emphasizes harmony in society, Taoism seeks unity with nature, and Buddhism turns inward to liberate the self from suffering (Yao, 2000).

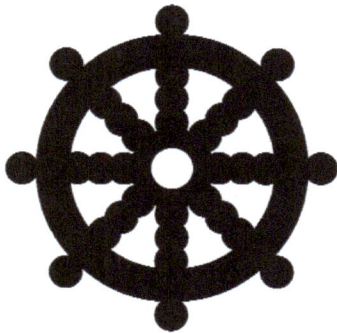 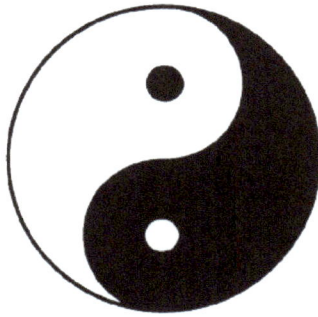 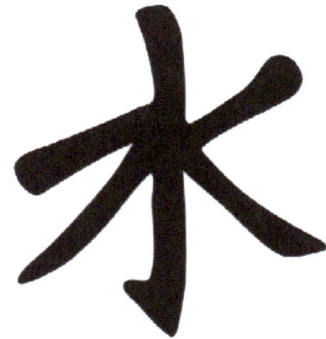

Buddhism   **Taoism**   **Confucianism**

Confucianism: The Order of Society

Founded by Confucius (Kong Fuzi) around the 5th century BCE, Confucianism centers on ethics, duty, and the cultivation of virtuous behavior within a structured society. It promotes familial piety (*xiao*), respect for hierarchy, and the importance of education and ritual (*li*) (Sontag, 1974). A Confucian life is guided by the roles of the parent, child, ruler, subject, and the fulfillment of these roles builds a just and orderly world. It teaches that virtue in leadership trickles down to the moral development of the people (Yao, 2000).

Taoism: Flowing with Nature

Rooted in the *Tao Te Ching* by Laozi, Taoism (or Daoism) champions spontaneity, simplicity, and harmony with the *Tao,* or the ineffable force that flows through all things (Laozi, trans. Mitchell, 1988). Rather than striving to control or fix the world, the Taoist seeks to align with the natural order through non-resistance (*wu wei*), letting go of ego, and observing the rhythms of nature. Taoism speaks to the middle-aged soul, or one who questions structure and seeks authenticity and fluidity in life (Kirkland, 2004).

Buddhism: Awakening the Inner Self

Brought to China from India around the 1st century CE, Buddhism introduced a new inwardness, emphasizing meditation, compassion, and release from suffering through the Eightfold Path (Harvey, 2013). The Buddhist focus is not on society or external alignment but on awakening. It teaches that all phenomena are impermanent, and that liberation comes not from control or flow, but from transcending attachment entirely (Mitchell, 2002). In this way, Buddhism serves the aging soul by contemplating, detaching, and seeking ultimate freedom.

Integration: A Balanced Life

In traditional Chinese thought, these three paths were not meant to compete but to complete one another. A person might live as:
- *a Confucian in the office*

- *a Taoist in the garden*

- *a Buddhist in solitude* (Yao, 2000).

Together, they offer a map to live wisely with integrity in society, harmony in nature, and peace within the soul.

References:

Sontag, F. (1974). Herbert Fingarette. Confucius—the Secular as Sacred. (Harper and Row, New York, 1972.). *Religious Studies*, *10*(2), 245–246. https://doi.org/10.1017/s0034412500007514

Harvey, P. (2012). *An introduction to Buddhism*. https://doi.org/10.1017/cbo9781139050531

Taoism: the Enduring tradition. (n.d.). Routledge & CRC Press. https://www.routledge.com/Taoism-The-Enduring-Tradition/Kirkland/p/book/9780415263221?utm_source=cjaffiliates&utm_medium=affiliates&cjevent=eeb2c6c93e3c11f083ff00cf0a82b820

Mitchell, S. (1988). Tao Te Ching. In *HARPERPERENNIAL MODERNCLASSICS*. HARPERPERENNIAL MODERNCLASSICS. https://ia800904.us.archive.org/20/items/taoteching-Stephen-Mitchell-translation-v9deoq/taoteching-Stephen-Mitchell-translation-v9deoq_text.pdf

Mitchell, D. W. (2002). *Buddhism: Introducing the Buddhist experience*. Oxford University Press.

Yao, X. (2000). *An introduction to confucianism*. https://doi.org/10.1017/cbo9780511800887

Philosophy or Religion?

Buddhism, Taoism, and Confucianism – a comparison of the 3 systems

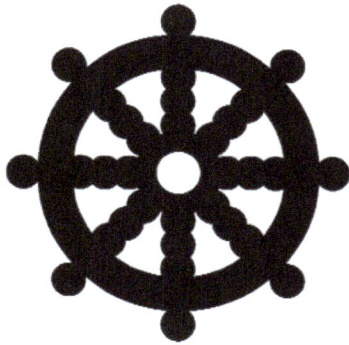

Buddhism

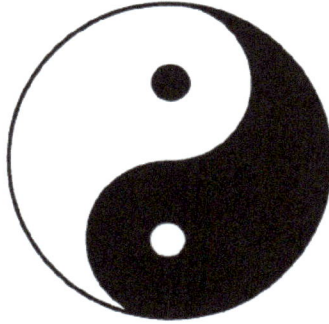

Taoism

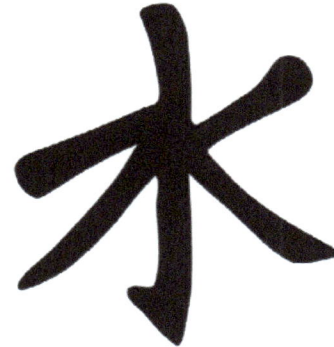

Confucianism

There is often debate as to what a philosophy is, versus that which is a religion. I have come to understand that there are fundamental differences between the two that are rooted in the goals, nature, and methods of each system. Religion seems to focus mostly on spiritual awareness through understanding and moral guidance, whereas philosophy embodies more broad topics such as science, logic, politics, and art. Philosophy looks to find truth in empirical and logical evidence, while religion usually accepts faith as valid evidence. Philosophy can be a broader, and more general field, where religion usually involves specific sets of beliefs and practices within a group. Philosophical aspects often appear within religions and consequently philosophical discussions about religious topics. The relationship between philosophy and religion can be complementary, where each can offer a unique perspective of human experience.

I write about this topic as I have found that individuals who have some type of relationship with either a life philosophy or religion, often have a stronger sense of purpose, meaning and gratitude beyond themselves. This often leads to a healthier and happier life. Also, association with a religion while aligning with a philosophical system need not be mutually exclusive to one another. In various parts of the world where people are free to worship and live as they may, one can be a Christian, Buddhist and Taoist if they so choose.

Buddhism, Taoism, and ***Confucianism*** are three of the most commonly practiced belief systems that are often labeled as philosophies, religions or even sometimes as both. The following is a summary of their origins and tenets:

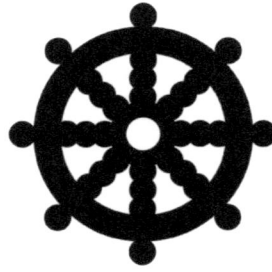

The 8-spoked wheel is often seen as a symbol for Buddhism.

Buddhism:
Origin:
- Buddhism was founded in the 6th century BCE by Buddha (563-483 BCE), also named Siddhartha Gautama, in ancient India which is today Nepal.

- Siddhartha was a prince who gave up his privileged life in order to better understand the nature of human suffering and to seek enlightenment or *nirvana*.

Core Tenets:
- The Four Noble Truths define the nature of suffering and a path to reduce its presence:

    - The Truth of Suffering (*Dukkha*): Buddhism acknowledges the existence of suffering and dissatisfaction in life. This suffering can be physical, emotional, or mental.

    - The Truth of the Cause of Suffering (*Samudaya*): Buddhism asserts that the root cause of suffering is craving or attachment (tanha) to things that are impermanent. This attachment leads to suffering because everything in the world is subject to change and eventual loss.

    - The Truth of the Cessation of Suffering (*Nirodha*): Buddhism teaches that it is possible to end suffering by letting go of attachment and craving. When one ceases to cling to impermanent things, suffering can be extinguished.

    - The Truth of the Path to the Cessation of Suffering (*Magga*): Buddhism offers a practical path called the Eightfold Path that leads to the cessation of suffering. This path consists of ethical and mental practices, such as right understanding, right intention, right speech, right action, right livelihood, right effort, right mindfulness, and right concentration.

- The Eight-fold Path provides a guide towards ethical and mental development needed to achieve enlightenment (Nirvana):

    - Right views

- Right aspirations
- Right speech
- Right conduct
- Right livelihood
- Right endeavor
- Right mindfulness
- Right meditation

Goal:
- The ultimate goal in Buddhism is to attain Nirvana, where there is a state of liberation from the continuous cycle of birth, death, and rebirth also known as *Samsara.*

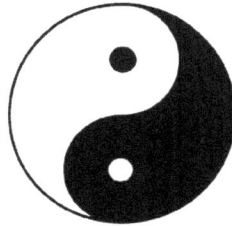

The *taijitsu* is often associated with Taoism and its concept of yin & yang.

Taoism:
Origin:
- Taoism, or sometimes *Daoism*, thought to have originated from Lao Tzu and his foundational text of the *Tao Te Ching* (The Way and Its Power), in China in the 6th century BCE.

Core Tenets:
- Main focus is upon trying to live in accordance to the *Tao* (the Way), which is thought to be the indefinable, fundamental force that unites all and everything in the universe.
- Another main principle is that of *Wu Wei* (effortless action), where one strives to live in harmony within the natural flow of the Tao rather than be subject to it.
- *Ying & yang* focuses upon the unity and duality inherent in all seeming opposites, such as: night-day, male-female, good-evil, positive-negative, etc.

Goal:

- Taoist philosophy strives to have the individual exist in a state of balance and harmony with the Tao, in order to align within the natural order of things, rather than imposing one's own will upon nature and the universe as a whole.

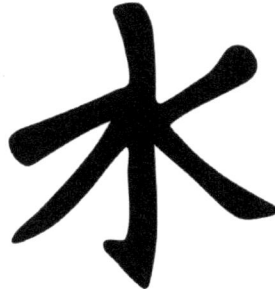

The Chinese character for water is often associated with Confucianism.

Confucianism:
Origin:
- Confucianism originated in China and was founded by Confucius (also known as Kong Fuzi) (551-479 BCE).

- Confucius was primarily concerned with understanding social order and its issues of ethics, morality, and the proper conduct of people living in society.

Core Tenets:
- Sacred texts of the *Wu Ching* (Five Classics) include the *I Ching* (Book of Changes), the *Lun-Yu* (The Analects)

- Emphasis is upon a moral code of:

  o *Li*: A code of moral/social conduct

  o *Jen*: Compassion/benevolence towards others

  o *Yi*: Righteousness

  o *Te*: Virtue

  o *Xiao*: Filial piety

- The importance of social harmony and the cultivation of moral character through education and self-cultivation.

- Emphasis upon the "Golden Rule" of "do not do unto others what you would not desire yourself."

Goal:

- Confucianism focuses upon establishing and maintaining a harmoniously functioning, well-ordered society through the virtuous persons who can fulfill their roles and responsibilities for the greater good of all.

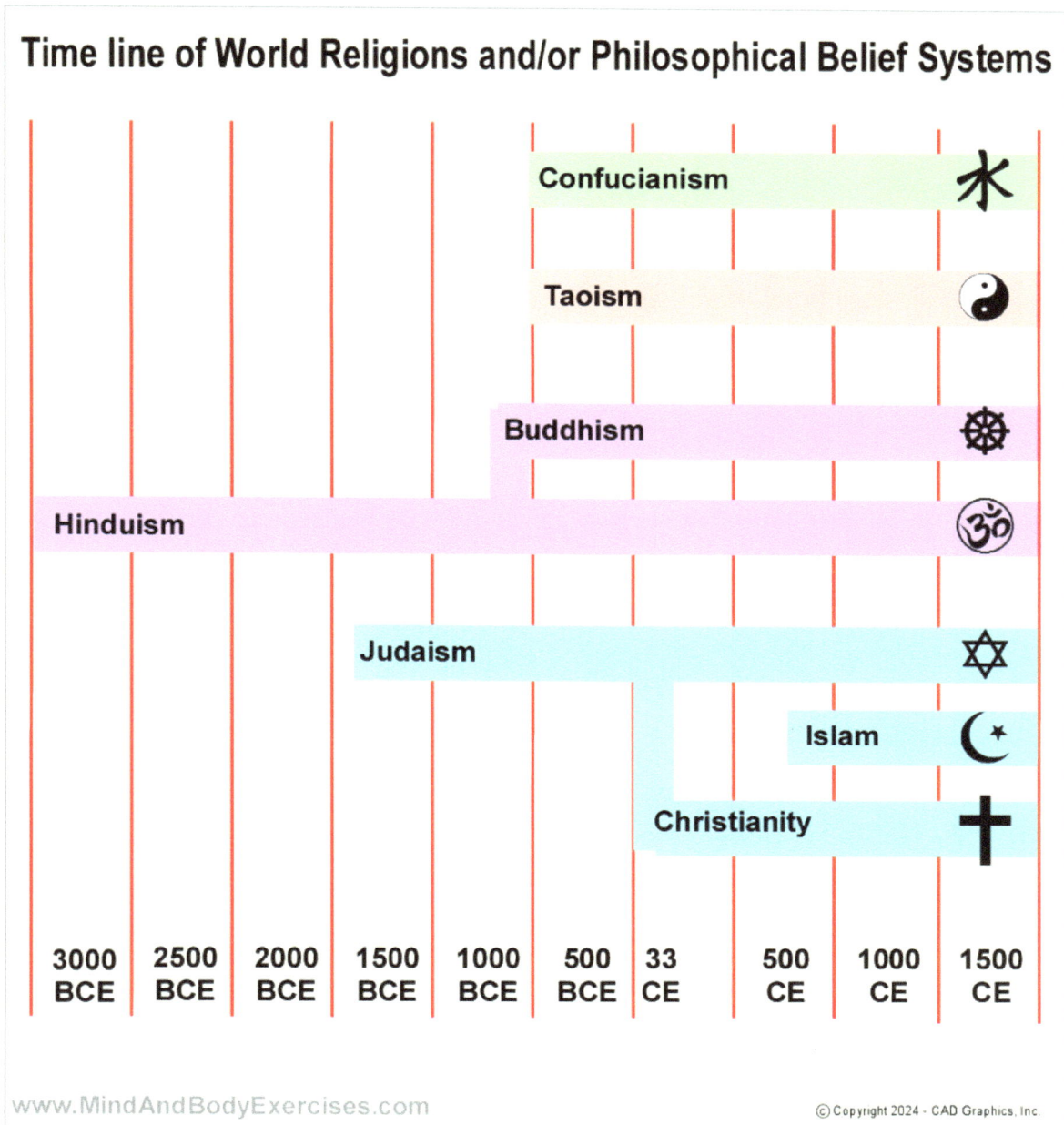

Time line of World Religions and/or Philosophical Belief Systems

Confucianism

Taoism

Buddhism

Hinduism

Judaism

Islam

Christianity

3000 BCE	2500 BCE	2000 BCE	1500 BCE	1000 BCE	500 BCE	33 CE	500 CE	1000 CE	1500 CE

From my research, there is no historical evidence that supports that the founders of Buddhism (Siddhartha Gautama), Taoism (Lao Tzu), and Confucianism (Confucius) had ever met one another, crossed paths or had interactions during their lifetimes. All three of these individuals lived in different times and places. Based upon the geographical distances as well as cultural differences between them, it is quite unlikely that these founders could have shared any direct experience or even knowledge of each other's existence.

These traditions often share some of the same philosophical ideas. Similarities in philosophical topics cultivated by these systems are most likely due to common exploration of universal ethical and existential questions during their times, rather than direct interactions or encounters among the founders. These systems do also have unique differences in their goals, teachings, methods, traditions, and approaches to life.

Comparisons between the three systems:

- **Basic Goals:**
  - Buddhism: understanding the self.
  - Taoism: understanding the self in relation to all else.
  - Confucianism: understanding the self and the relationship to society.

- **Geographic Origins:**
  - Buddhism: India
  - Taoism: China
  - Confucianism: China

- **Founders:**
  - Buddhism: Siddhartha Gautama (Buddha)
  - Taoism: Often associated with Lao Tzu
  - Confucianism: Confucius

- **Central Concepts:**
  - Buddhism: Four Noble Truths, Eightfold Path, nirvana
  - Taoism: Tao, wu wei, yin & yang
  - Confucianism: Li, Jen, Te, Yi, Xiao

- **Ultimate Goal:**
  - Buddhism: Nirvana
  - Taoism: Harmony with the Tao
  - Confucianism: Social harmony through moral character and cultivation

- **Perspective on Life:**
  - Buddhism: reduce suffering, detach from desires.
  - Taoism: alignment and harmony with the Tao
  - Confucianism: ethical conduct and social responsibilities

Cultural and Ethical Considerations in Mind-Body Medicine

I have previously discussed herbs and some of the ways that people self-prescribe with no real education in herbs, or their consumption based upon individual constitution rather than general acceptance of an herb as being healthy for all. I see this as taking the sweet of the benefits from these herbs but not taking the sour or learning the background or implications of using particular herbs. Basically, taking the culture at a superficial level for personal gain – cultural appropriation.

Anise
The overconsumption can affect the performance of birth control medication.

Cinnamon
It should be avoided by those who are taking prescribed blood thinners or due to undergo surgery.

Boldo and Cinnamon
In large doses, these herbs can exacerbate the effects of hepatotoxic drugs.

Eucalyptus
In medicinal doses, it can intensify the effects of diabetes drugs.

St. John's wort
If consumed alongside antidepressants, this herb can cause serotonin syndrome.

10 Facts About Medicinal Herbs and Prescription Drugs

Ginger
It contains chemicals that can aggravate the effects of diabetes medication.

Grapefruit
When consumed with certain statins, it can trigger adverse reactions.

Lemon Balm
Avoid consumption simultaneously with CNS depressants.

Coffee
Caffeine accompanying ephedrine can induce arrhythmia or a heart attack.

Lavender
This herb should not be administered to those who are taking sedative drugs.

www.herbazest.com

https://www.herbazest.com/wellness-articles/10-facts-about-medicinal-herbs-and-prescription-drugs

Watering-down or cultural exploitation of yoga is an easy target as a big player in this controversial topic. Meditation practices have become diluted from spiritual or self-awareness practices from yoga and its relative qigong counterpart. With more attention towards stress management through mindfulness and mindful breathing or breathwork, many will have an attraction towards these practices without having any spiritual connection to these methods.

All You Can Attend Exercise Buffet

- yoga   - tai chi

- pilates   - qigong

- meditation - cardio kung fu

99¢ per person, no sharing please

Living in this time of great technological advances and access to an almost unlimited supply of online information for healthcare and almost every other topic, has its own issues of pros and cons. With great knowledge, comes great responsibility or a similar cliché from pop-culture. A large percentage of people in the US have access to watch YouTube or other online outlets to view and learn about acupuncture and other Traditional Chinese Medicine methods, massage, yoga, Ayurveda and many other worldwide traditional mind and body practices.

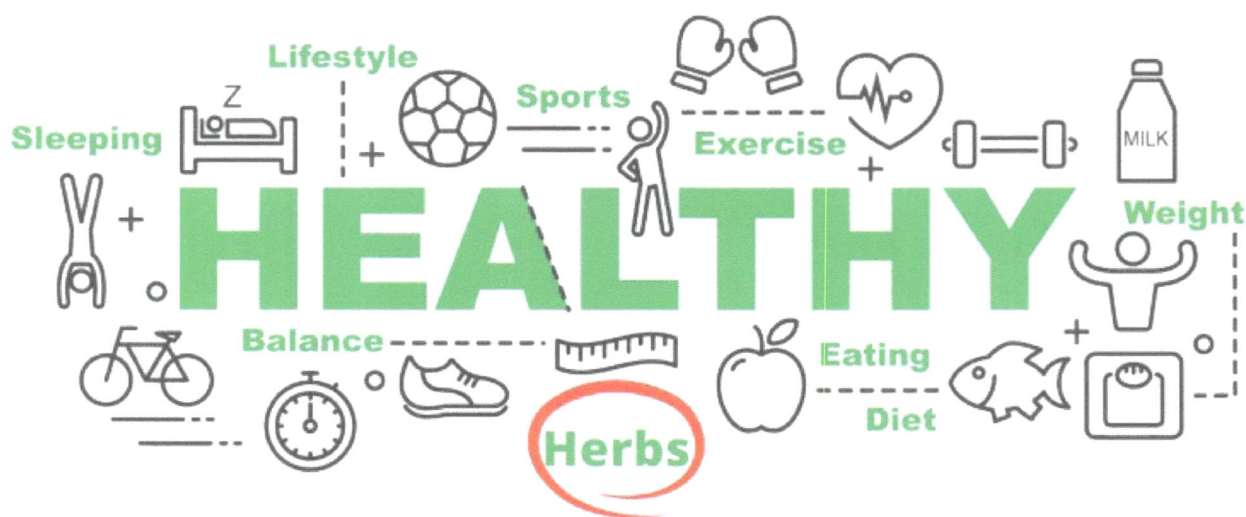

https://www.deanlong.io/blog/herb-supplements-boosting-mens-energy-performance-in-sports-and-sex

With this access many can not only become more knowledgeable but can also often self-prescribe, self-diagnose, and self-administer many of these methods with no real academic nor clinical education. Where we may enjoy the benefits of this access, we must realize that some will abuse this knowledge or interpret it incorrectly and use it themselves or pass it on to others, in the hope of helping others or profiting for their own benefit. If qualified, educated people post this knowledge and information for others to view and/or study, how can some people complain that others are then using this knowledge as cultural appropriation? With most freedoms, there is a cost in order to have and maintain them.

References:

Eichhorn, T., Greten, H. J., & Efferth, T. (2011). Self-medication with nutritional supplements and herbal over-thecounter products. Natural Products and Bioprospecting, 1(2), 62–70. https://doi.org/10.1007/s13659-011-0029-1

https://www.ayurvedanama.org/articles/2021/3/18/the-dangers-of-self-medicating-with-herbs

https://www.herbazest.com/wellness-articles/10-facts-about-medicinal-herbs-and-prescription-drugs

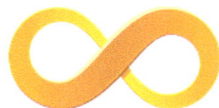

True, Right, and Correct

I have engaged in quite a few discussions regarding "truth" with others over my years. I have learned from my observations and in particular that "kind words are seldom true; true words are seldom kind". True words can be uncomfortable or even painful for the speaker as well as the recipient. But like you stated, being a desirable dinner guest might not be your goal.

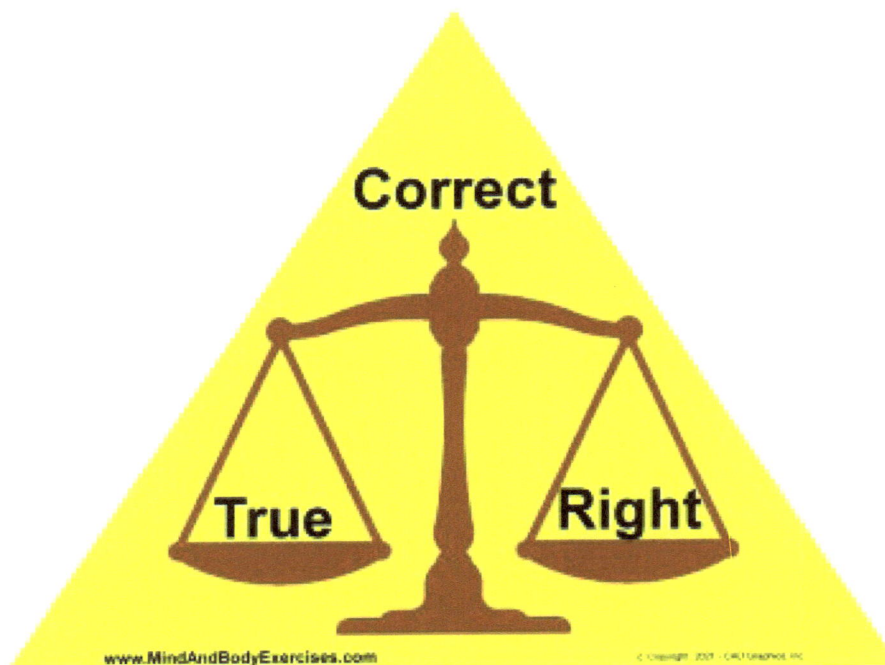

I was taught from my experiences within martial arts and its background in Taoism, Buddhism and Confucianism, the concept of balancing true, right and correct. We often find ourselves trying to balance ourselves between what is true, right or correct for any given situation and particular circumstances for any specific time and place. What was true yesterday may not be today. What is appropriate in one setting, may not be for another. If we tell the truth to a young child about birth, murder, drugs and other complex subjects, before their understanding is appropriate, it may cause damage to their perspectives for years to come. However, if we do what we feel is right and maybe shield them from reality, this too may cause potential issues down the road. Correct, however, is the balance we seek to find between true and right. So, in other words, I do not think the truth is totally absolute and appropriate for all situations.

Wisdom is a recipe of knowledge and experience obtained over time (age) allowing one to differentiate when the correct timing is to react or not to react. When to do, when not to do. Coming up to a stop sign, you really don't care to stop your vehicle (your true feeling) but you do because it is the right action (the law) to stop. If a blaring fire engine were to suddenly appear in your rear-view mirror, you might choose to move through the intersection and to a space clear of the oncoming 370,000 pounds of moving metal and water (correct action for this situation).

In an age dominated by speed, data, and polarization, the need for wise decision-making has never been greater. While traditional critical thinking focuses on logic and evidence, it often omits other dimensions of human understanding, such as authenticity, ethics, and contextual appropriateness. The "True, Right, and Correct" framework expands critical thinking into a multidimensional model that integrates intellectual rigor with moral clarity and practical wisdom.

This model draws from philosophical reasoning, spiritual awareness, and functional discernment to offer a more holistic approach to evaluating choices, actions, and beliefs.

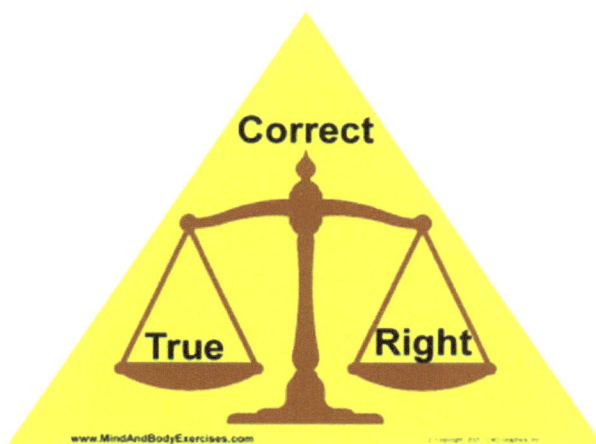

Expanding Critical Thinking: A Holistic Triad

Critical thinking is often defined as the ability to analyze, evaluate, and synthesize information in order to form reasoned judgments. It relies on logic, evidence, skepticism, and reasoning. However, while these tools are necessary, they are not always sufficient.

The "True, Right, and Correct" framework offers a layered upgrade to conventional critical thinking:

Aspect	Conventional Critical Thinking	True-Right-Correct Framework
Logic	Essential	Integrated within "Right"
Ethics	Optional or minimal	Central under "True"
Authenticity	Rarely addressed	Essential under "True"
Intuition/Conscience	Often ignored	Embraced within "True" and "Right"
Functional Aptness	Sometimes included	Core under "Correct"

Overview of the Two-lens Model

The framework is visualized as a Venn diagram with two intersecting circles and the portion that overlaps to form a third zone:

- **TRUE** – Inner authenticity and alignment with reality

- **RIGHT** – Moral integrity and ethical discernment

- **CORRECT** – Balance of technical soundness and contextual precision

Where these two elements intersect is the "zone of wise action."

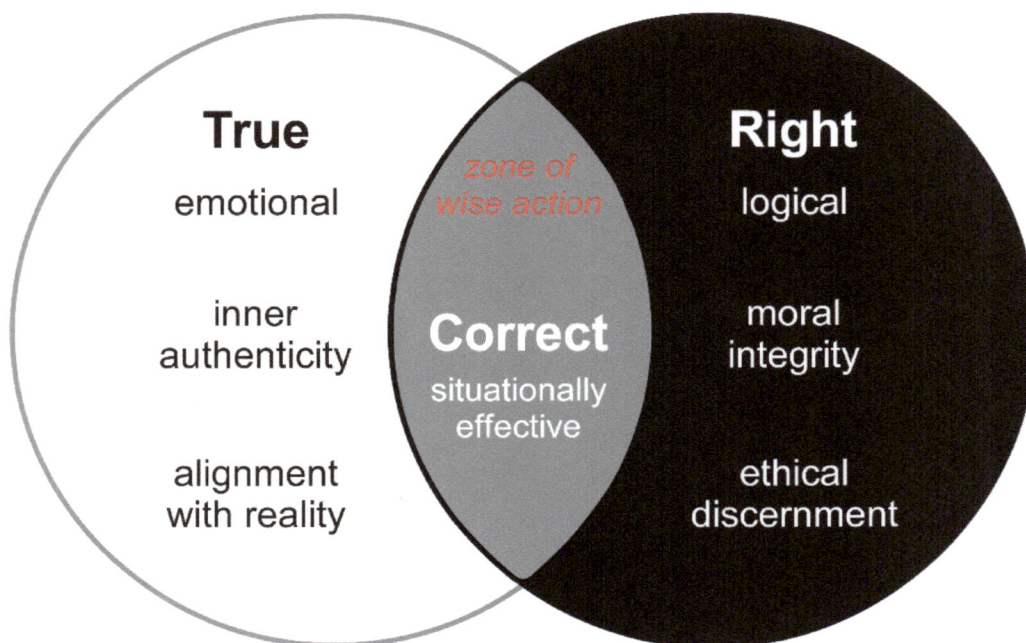

True
emotional
zone of wise action
logical
Right
inner
authenticity
Correct
situationally
effective
moral
integrity
alignment
with reality
ethical
discernment

1. TRUE: Alignment with Reality and Authenticity
- **Definition**: What aligns with one's inner values, lived experience, or observable truth

- **Includes**: Self-awareness, factual clarity, personal integrity, intuitive knowing

- **Example**: Expressing a difficult truth even when it's unpopular

Critical Thinking Link: Encourages self-honesty and questions personal assumptions

Reflection Questions:
- Am I being honest with myself and others?

- Is this based on what is real or what is assumed?

- Does this reflect my core values and lived experiences?

2. RIGHT: Moral and Ethical Discernment
- **Definition**: What is just, compassionate, and beneficial from a moral perspective

- **Includes**: Fairness, empathy, justice, long-term benefit to others

- **Example**: Choosing not to exploit a legal loophole because it harms others

Critical Thinking Link: Adds an ethical filter to decisions that might otherwise be purely strategic

Reflection Questions:
- Is this action fair and just?

- Would I consider this acceptable if done to me?

- Does this honor both the letter and spirit of the greater good?

3. CORRECT: The Balance of Functional Precision and Situational Appropriateness
- **Definition**: What is technically accurate, logically coherent, and situationally effective

- **Includes**: Evidence-based reasoning, timing, execution, contextual fit

- **Example**: Using the correct communication method for sensitive feedback

Critical Thinking Link: Embeds the core tools of analysis, logic, and evidence evaluation

Reflection Questions:
- Is this the best balance between true and right, that can serve the most involved?

- Is this method sound and supported by facts?

- Am I choosing the most effective way to act or express this?

- Is it appropriate for this time, place, and audience?

Applications in Teaching and Practice This framework serves as a compass for ethical leadership, personal reflection, and integrative education:
- **In classrooms**: Pairing logic with ethics and introspection

- **In leadership**: Building trust through aligned, values-driven decisions

- **In personal growth**: Assessing decisions using a whole-self model

- **In debate and conflict**: Seeking understanding through multiple lenses

Teaching Module Activities

1. **Case Study Analysis** – Analyze real-world dilemmas from all three perspectives

2. **Personal Journaling** – Reflect on a difficult decision using the lens of true, right, and correct

3. **Group Debates** – Discuss how outcomes shift when one element is missing

4. **Visual Mapping** – Place actions on a Venn diagram to assess alignment

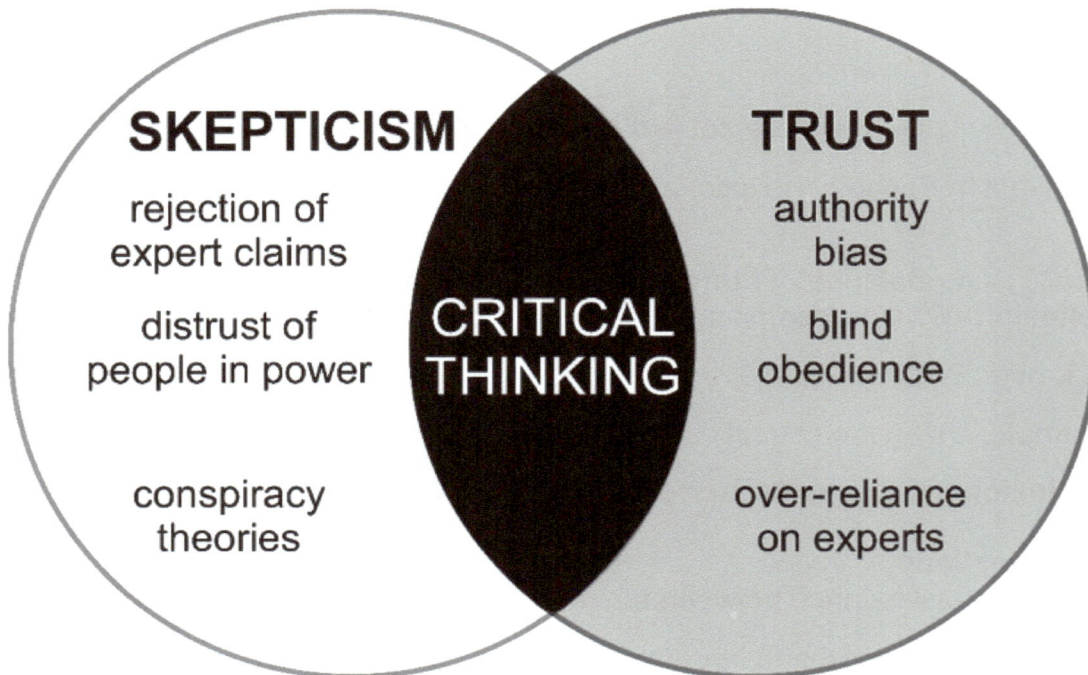

SKEPTICISM
rejection of expert claims

distrust of people in power

conspiracy theories

CRITICAL THINKING

TRUST
authority bias

blind obedience

over-reliance on experts

Conclusion The "True, Right, and Correct" framework expands critical thinking into a richer, more human-centered process. It challenges individuals not just to think better, but to *live* and *act* more wisely through authenticity, ethical clarity, and contextual intelligence. In doing so, it reclaims critical thinking not only as a cognitive skill, but as a moral and spiritual practice.

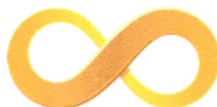

Seek the Right Teacher

If you need to improve your balance, seek someone who can demonstrate balance.

If you need to improve your bone strength, seek someone who can demonstrate strength in their bones.

If you need to strengthen and/or improve flexibility in your spine, seek someone who can demonstrate how to do so.

Move beyond thinking that your health and well-being are someone else's responsibility. Be more active, eat healthier, sleep better, stress less – these are the key components to maintaining a strong immune system.

Across time and cultures, the greatest spiritual teachers have emphasized simplicity, humility, and inner transformation. Yet, paradoxically, the institutions that grow around these teachings often accumulate material wealth, political power, and ego-driven prestige.

Christianity, Buddhism, Hinduism, Islam, all at their core, advocate for the shedding of worldly attachments. Yet many of their largest institutions exhibit the very materialism and hierarchy their founders warned against. In light of today's cultural unrest, consumerism, and spiritual seeking, these contradictions deserve closer reflection.

A Humble Beginning

Jesus of Nazareth lived with radical humility. His birth in a manger (Luke 2:7, New International Version [NIV]), his itinerant lifestyle (*"the Son of Man has no place to lay his head,"* Luke 9:58, NIV), and his repeated critiques of religious legalism (Matthew 23:1–28, NIV) demonstrate a clear rejection of material power and ritualized pretense.
He warned against storing up treasures on earth, urging people instead to seek spiritual treasures (Matthew 6:19–21, NIV). His message was direct: inner transformation and compassion mattered more than public ritual or personal gain.

And yet, centuries later, the Roman Catholic Church emerged from the very empire that crucified him, to became one of the wealthiest and most ritualized institutions in human history (MacCulloch, 2011).

A Universal Paradox

This irony is not exclusive to Christianity. It is a universal pattern across major belief systems:

- **Buddhism**: Siddhartha Gautama, the Buddha, renounced his royal status to seek enlightenment through simplicity and meditation. His core teaching of the elimination of craving and attachment became institutionalized into monasteries and sects, some of which, over centuries, accumulated wealth, political influence, and hierarchical authority (Lopez, 2001).

- **Hinduism**: Early Vedic teachings stressed detachment from material life through paths like *Jnana* (knowledge) and *Bhakti* (devotion). Yet, sprawling temple complexes, priestly hierarchies, and caste structures often mirrored societal materialism and status-seeking (Flood, 1996).

- **Islam**: The Prophet Muhammad lived simply, called for humility, and emphasized equality among believers. Yet throughout history, caliphates and modern regimes alike have at times entangled faith with vast political and material ambitions (Esposito, 1998).

Again and again, humanity seems to be drawn to codify spiritual simplicity into worldly complexity.

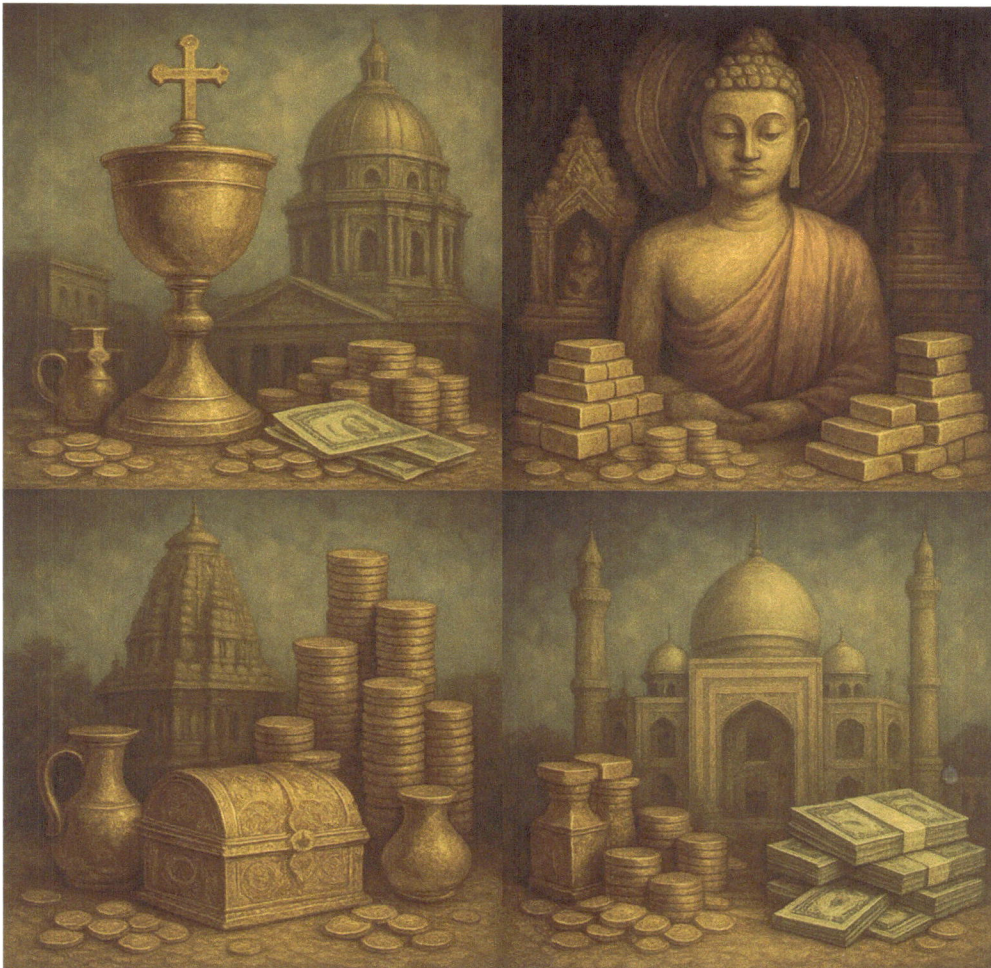

Why Does This Happen?

From a psychological and sociological standpoint, this paradox might stem from natural human tendencies:

- **Desire for Security**: Spiritual communities often accumulate resources to protect their teachings and communities from external threats.

- **Institutionalization**: Movements grow into organizations, and organizations seek stability, leading to bureaucracy and hierarchy.

- **Human Ego**: Even with the best intentions, individuals and groups may seek recognition, authority, and influence, contradicting the original teachings.

As the Tao Te Ching observes, *"The higher the structure, the farther from the Way"* (Laozi, trans. Mitchell, 1988).

Cultural Relevance Today

Today's society, riddled with consumerism, curated self-images, and institutional distrust, mirrors these spiritual paradoxes. Many seekers are disillusioned with religious structures not because they reject faith, but because they crave *authenticity*.

Holistic health practitioners recognize that wellness is found in true balance of mind, body, and spirit, and requires stripping away external noise and realigning with essential truths. It's not in grandeur but in simplicity that healing often occurs. The example of figures like Jesus, Buddha, and Muhammad calls us back not to ritualized identity, but to the living essence of humility, compassion, and conscious living.

A Personal Reflection

This reflection isn't a condemnation of all spiritual institutions. Rather, it is a call to vigilance:
- Are we aligning with the heart of spiritual wisdom or merely its outer forms?

- Are we living simply, authentically, and compassionately, or becoming entangled in ego, status, and recognition?

As individuals seeking holistic well-being, we are invited to live in *the spirit* rather than merely follow *the form*.

Spiritual maturity requires discernment and choosing the inward journey over external display, whether in religion, health, or daily life.

References:

Esposito, J. L. (1998). *Islam: The straight path* (3rd ed.). Oxford University Press.

Flood, G. (1996). *An introduction to Hinduism*. Cambridge University Press.

Lopez, D. S., Jr. (2001). *THE STORY OF BUDDHISM*. HarperSanFrancisco. http://www.chanreads.org/wp-content/uploads/2022/09/The-Story-of-Buddhism-A-Concise-Guide-to-Its-History-Teachings-Donald-S.-Lopez-Jr.-chanreads.org_.pdf

MacCulloch, D. (2011). *Christianity: The first three thousand years*. Penguin Books.

Mitchell, S. (Trans.). (1988). *Tao Te Ching* (Lao Tzu). Harper & Row.

The Holy Bible, New International Version. (2011). Biblica, Inc. (Original work published 1978)

Gong De Wei Shen

The term **Gong De Wei Shen** (功德为神) could loosely be interpreted as "acquiring karmic merit for spiritual elevation or connection to the divine." It's a phrase that might not appear in ancient texts directly but captures the concept of dedicating good deeds or spiritual work to elevate one's spiritual state, aligning with Chinese philosophies of moral virtue influencing one's spiritual development. **Gong De Wei Shen** is indeed rooted in Chinese philosophical and spiritual traditions, though the exact expression isn't commonly cited. I will break it down to the best of my understanding:

1. **Gong (功):** This translates to merit, achievement, accomplishment, or work.

2. **Gong de (功德):** This translates to "merit" or "karmic merit" or virtuous deeds as used in Buddhist and Taoist traditions in the sense of virtue accumulated through good deeds and moral actions of generosity and compassion towards others. In traditional Chinese thought and in Buddhism, *gong de* is the spiritual merit or positive karma gained through altruistic actions, spiritual practice, and moral conduct. These merits are believed to contribute to spiritual growth and favorable outcomes in this life or future lives

3. **Wei (为)**: This can mean "for" or "as" in this context, often used to imply that the merit serves or benefits something.

4. **Shen 神 :** This translates to "spirit" or "divine" and can suggest a higher spiritual state or connection with the divine.

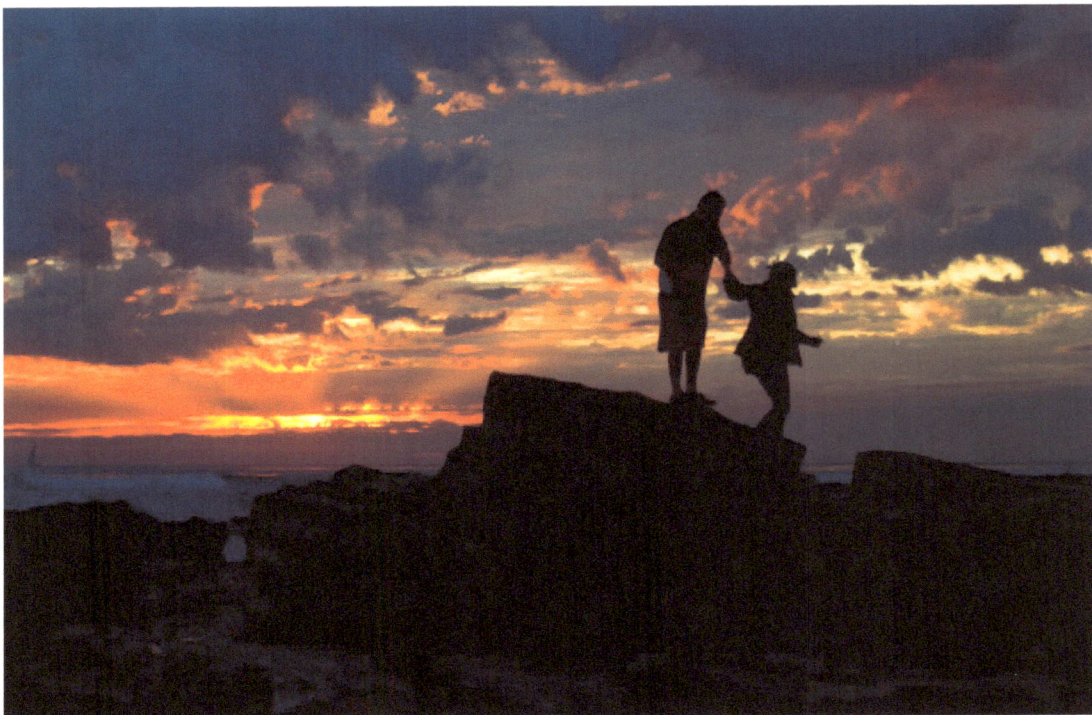

While *gong de wei shen*, itself isn't a phrase widely cited in ancient texts, some numerous classical works and studies delve into the related concepts of *gong de* (karmic merit), the role of *shen* (spirit or divine), and the accumulation of spiritual merit through virtuous actions. Here are some references that explore these themes:

1. **Dao De Jing (Tao Te Ching)** by Lao Tzui: One of the foundational texts of Daoism, the *Dao De Jing* discusses concepts of virtue (*de*, 德) and alignment with the *Dao* (道) as a path to spiritual harmony. While it may not explicitly use *gong de*, it emphasizes the moral conduct and inner qualities that create harmony with the universe.

2. **The Avatamsaka Sutra (Huayan Sutra)**: In Mahayana Buddhism, which has heavily influenced Chinese thought, the *Avatamsaka Sutra* (华严经, *Huayan Jing*) explores the concept of *merit* (功德, *gong de*) in spiritual practice and its effect on one's path toward enlightenment. This text connects good deeds and moral actions with spiritual progression.

3. **The Book of Changes (I Ching)**: Though more symbolic, the *I Ching* reflects on the harmony between human actions and spiritual forces, suggesting that righteous behavior impacts one's fate and connection with higher powers.

4. **Zhuangzi**: This Daoist text, attributed to the philosopher Zhuang Zhou, explores spiritual transformation and the concept of *shen* as something cultivated through inner clarity and virtue.

The concepts of 功德 (gong de, karmic merit) and 神修 (shen xiu, spiritual cultivation) are deeply relevant to everyday life, even for those who don't actively follow Taoist or Buddhist traditions. Here's why they can be important:

1. Actions Shape Our Lives and Mindset

Every small act of kindness, generosity, or ethical behavior accumulates *gong de* not just in a spiritual sense but in how it influences your relationships, reputation, and self-perception. Helping a friend, being honest in business, or treating people with respect builds trust and goodwill, which can often return in unexpected ways.

Spiritual wellness is...

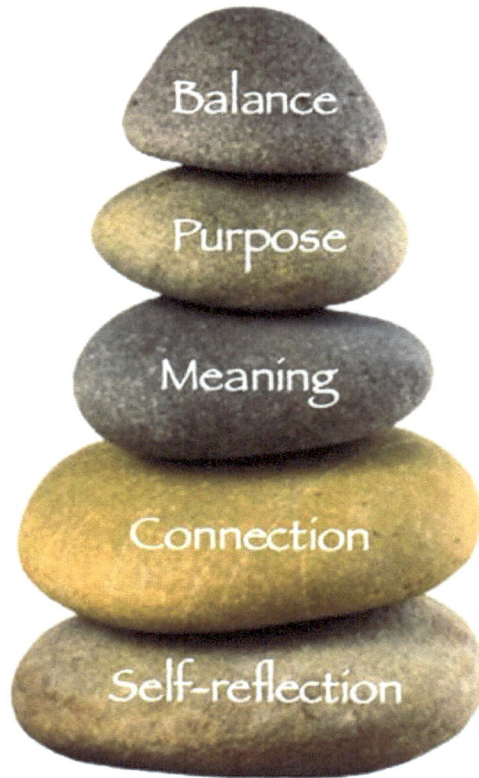

Balance

Purpose

Meaning

Connection

Self-reflection

2. Inner Peace Comes from Spiritual Awareness

Spiritual cultivation (*shen xiu*) isn't about being religious, but rather developing self-awareness, clarity, and emotional balance. In daily life, this may be practiced as:

- Pausing before reacting negatively in a stressful situation.

- Practicing mindfulness or gratitude to reduce anxiety.

- Seeking wisdom in challenges rather than reacting impulsively.

3. Good Energy Attracts Good Outcomes

Many people unconsciously follow the idea of karma or energetic reciprocity. When you consistently act with integrity and positive intention, life tends to reflect that back. We sometimes call this *"what goes around, comes around."* This is why some who choose to cultivate *gong de* often experience more fulfilling relationships, career success, and personal growth.

4. Resilience in Hard Times

Practicing *gong de* and *shen xiu* helps you build inner strength. When facing setbacks, those who have cultivated patience, kindness, and wisdom may be better equipped to manage challenges with grace, rather than feeling like a victim of circumstances.

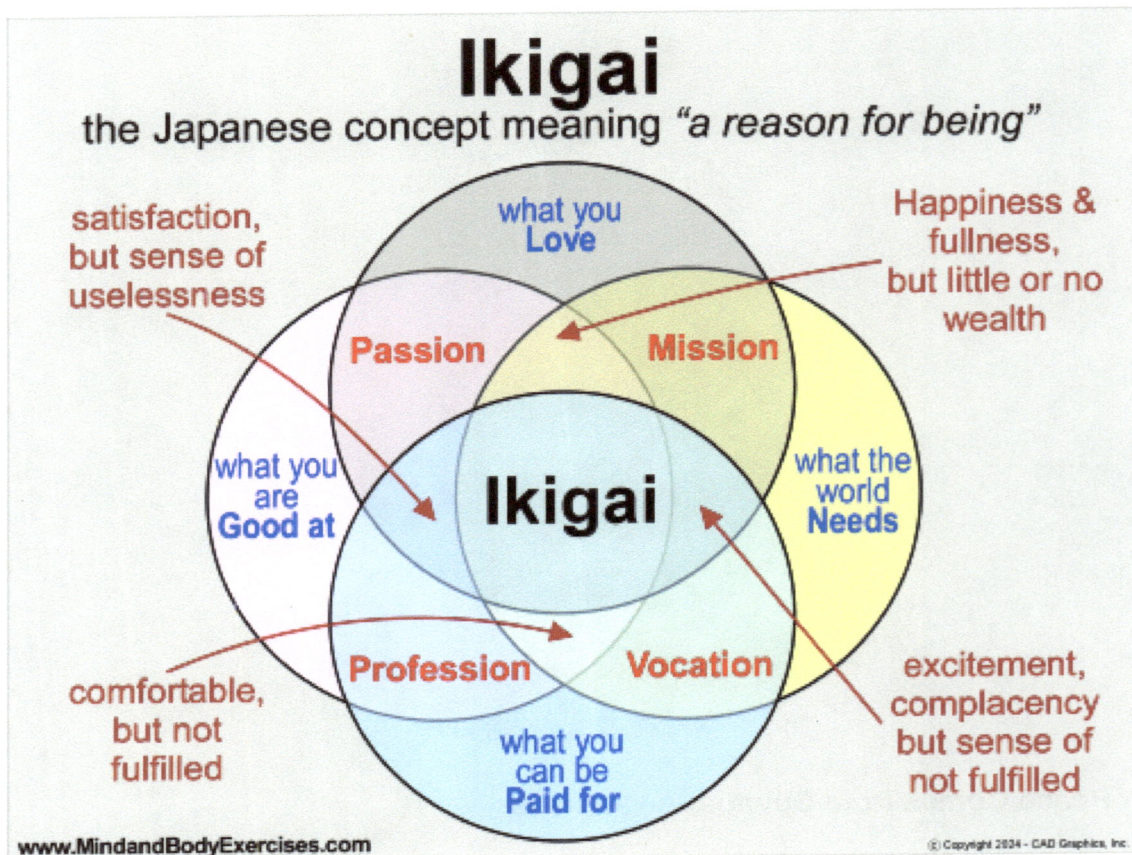

Ikigai
the Japanese concept meaning *"a reason for being"*

satisfaction, but sense of uselessness

Happiness & fullness, but little or no wealth

what you **Love**

Passion   **Mission**

what you are **Good at**   **Ikigai**   what the world **Needs**

Profession   **Vocation**

comfortable, but not fulfilled

what you can be **Paid for**

excitement, complacency but sense of not fulfilled

www.MindandBodyExercises.com   © Copyright 2024 - CAD Graphics, Inc.

5. A Sense of Purpose

Beyond material success, many people seek meaning in their daily lives. The Japanese term of ***Ikigai*** embodies the concept of meaning, purpose along with other aspects of passion and profession.. Spiritual cultivation (*shen xiu*) can provide a sense of meaning or purpose, whether through meditation, learning, creative expression, or simply striving to be a better person.

In Summary

These aren't just ancient ideas, but rather practical tools for striving to live a more peaceful, balanced, and fulfilling life. By cultivating merit (*gong de*) and refining your inner spirit (*shen xiu*), one may naturally create a more harmonious life, both for themselves and those around them.

Become the Diamond, Leave the Coal Behind

Humans are like a lump of coal (or carbon), where if put under enough pressure, we may transform into a diamond. I understand that it takes many years, perhaps millions of years, for this transformation to happen. As humans we have only about 70-80 years on average to make our transformation come about, so best to start as soon as possible. I speak of this diamond metaphorically, in regard to each of us being on our own journey to find purpose and meaning in our lives. The diamond is what emerges from the dark and dirty coal, as we strive to find the inner genius, beauty, perfection and acceptance within ourselves.

We all have our own unique set of circumstances with relative trials and tribulations. How we manage these issues are key to our health and happiness. Managing our thoughts, emotions and actions can often be attained from managing our physical body through exercise and deliberate wellness and fitness methods. Qigong (yoga), tai chi, meditation and other methods can offer lifelong benefits to the mind, body and spirit. These practices are paths to become your diamond from the rough of the world.

"Diamond"
is a chunk of coal
that did well under pressure

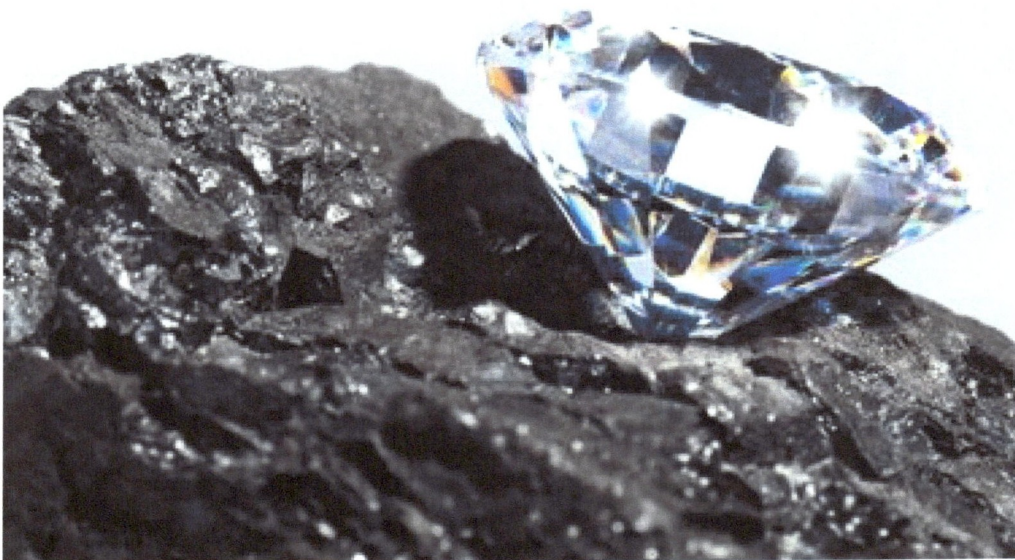

- Henry Kissinger

The process of transforming coal into a diamond takes an incredibly long time—millions to billions of years. Both coal and diamonds are made up of carbon, but the key difference lies in their formation and the conditions under which they are created.

Coal forms from plant material that accumulates in swampy environments over millions of years. Through the process of burial and geological transformation, the organic material undergoes compaction and chemical changes, resulting in the formation of coal. This process typically takes millions of years.

On the other hand, diamonds are formed deep within the Earth's mantle, where high pressure and temperature conditions exist. These conditions cause carbon atoms to arrange in a crystal lattice structure, forming diamonds. This process occurs at depths of around 150 to 200 kilometers (93 to 124 miles) and requires immense pressure and temperatures of approximately 1,000 to 1,300 degrees Celsius (1,832 to 2,372 degrees Fahrenheit). The time required for diamond formation can range from hundreds of millions to billions of years.

Therefore, the transformation of coal into a diamond is an extremely slow and geologically long process, occurring over millions to billions of years under specific conditions deep within the Earth.

Life is a challenge. Nothing worth achieving comes for free. Gifts and rewards are most valuable when earned. Change your coal into diamonds.

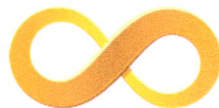

The Dunning-Kruger Effect

High

Confidence

Peak of Enthusiasm
- incompetent's hubris
- "I know it all"

Plateau of Sustainability

- "Now I get it"
- "This is still difficult, but worth it"

Valley of Despair
- "I may be wrong"
- "There is more to this"

- "I might be starting to understand"
- "This is difficult"

Slope of Enlightenment

High

Low

Competence - Knowledge - Experience

| enthusiasm | despair | enlightenment | sustainability |

www.MindAndBodyExercises.com

© Copyright 2024 - CAD Graphics, Inc.

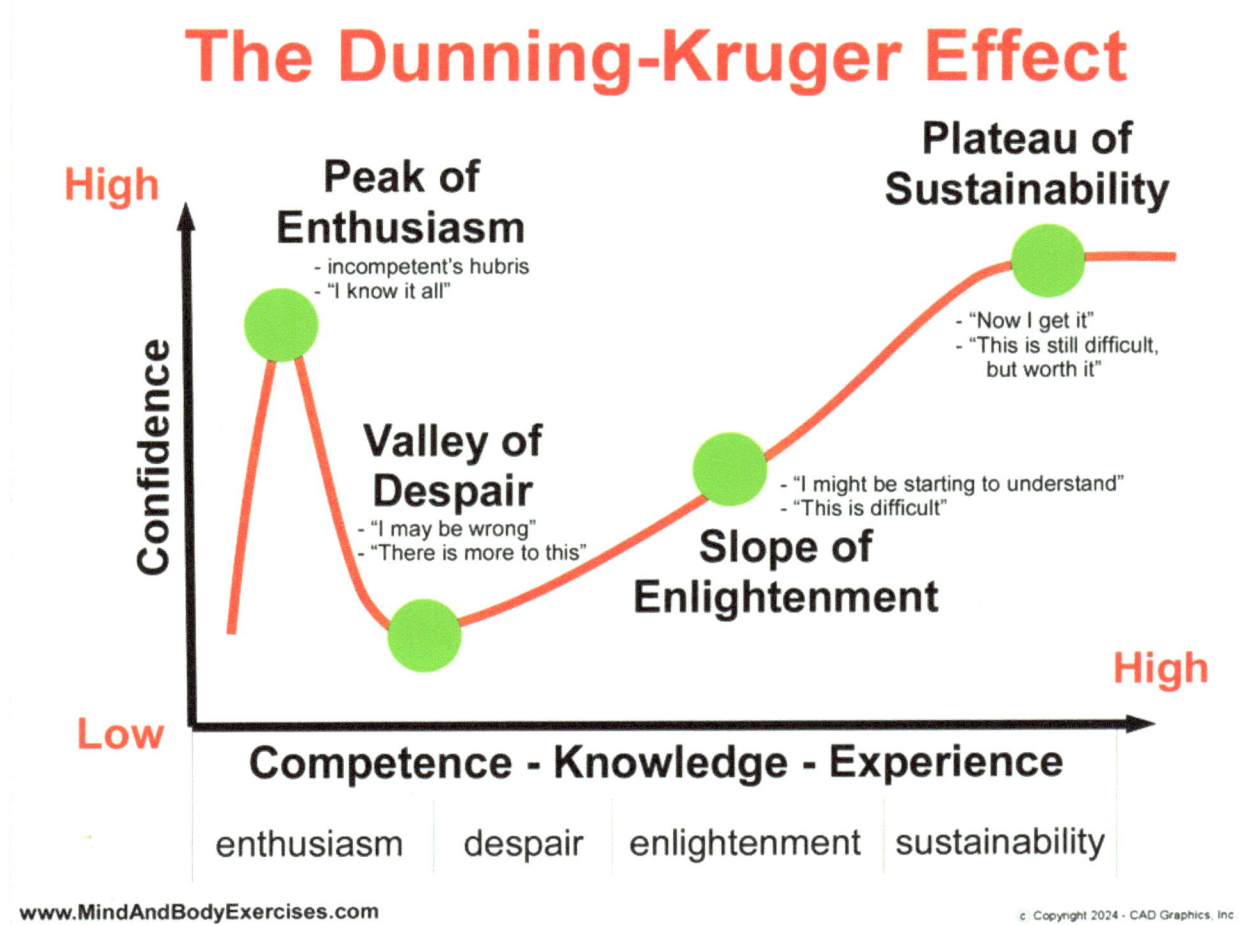

The Dunning-Kruger effect was theorized by psychologists David Dunning and Justin Kruger in a 1999 study. They proposed that there is a cognitive bias where individuals with knowledge or ability within a specific area have a propensity to overestimate their own competence in a particular field. This overestimation may come about due to a lack of the necessary metacognitive skills to accurately determine their own competence.

A common phrase used to summarize this phenomenon is that of *"they don't know, what they don't know."* This effect may be seen in examples of recent high school or college graduates who sometimes express a type of hubris, where they believe that they are intellectually superior to others. Expecting parents sometimes experience this effect where before their child is born, they have delusions of what type of parents they will be. "My kids won't get away with that," "I won't be doing that with my children," or maybe prejudging other parents in how they choose to raise their kids. Once their children are born, new parents might soon realize that parenting is much more complex and difficult than what they first believed.

Know-it-All

Conversely, those individuals who are highly knowledgeable or skilled in a particular field often underestimate their own competence. This underestimation may manifest because some individuals assume that challenges or projects that are easy for them may also be easy for most others. Well-seasoned individuals in any particular field of knowledge, skill, or ability often gain much wisdom from experience, adaptation, and application of their specific skill set. For some people, this is also highly humbling as the individual realizes that the more someone knows, they ironically recognize that there is so much more to learn.

The Dunning-Kruger effect can be summarized into four key stages:

1. **Incompetence and Confidence:** Individuals possessing low skill levels or knowledge may fail to acknowledge their lack of skill, leading to inflated self-assessments and high confidence.

2. **Awareness of Incompetence:** Once an individual acquires more knowledge and experience, they may start to become more aware of their own incompetence, which in turn leads to a further decrease in confidence.

3. **Competence along with Cautious Confidence:** With further experience, practice, and learning, individuals begin to develop true competence. As their confidence begins to increase again, they can more accurately showcase their abilities.

4. **Mastery with Modesty:** More highly skilled individuals will often acknowledge the complexities of a particular domain and realize how much they still don't know. This awareness can lead to modesty or humbleness about their abilities, despite the individual being highly competent in their specific field.

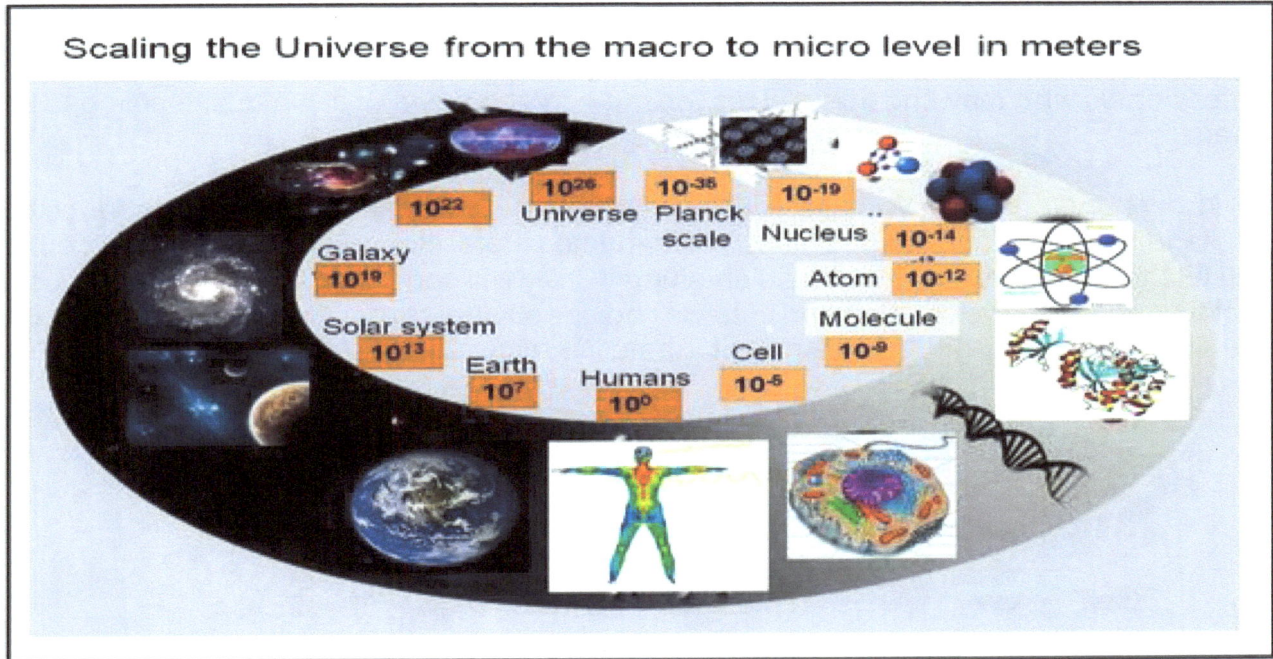

Scaling the Universe from the macro to micro level in meters

The Dunning-Kruger effect highlights the importance of seeking self-awareness and striving to continue to learn new things. It proposes that improving one's metacognitive skills, such as the ability to self-assess one's own knowledge and performance accurately can help minimize the effect.

In summary, the Dunning-Kruger effect is a cognitive bias where individuals with low knowledge, ability, or competence in a specific area may overestimate their own skill level. On the other hand, people with a high competence in a particular field often underestimate their relative ability. This may occur due to the same skills that contribute to competence also needed to recognize competence, leading to a disconnect between self-assessment and actual ability.

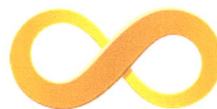

Abundance

You can only give out what you yourself have an abundance of.

Over the years, I have learned a bit about energetics from my massage therapists as well as my martial arts and qigong teachers. During a massage, the practitioner expends physical effort and mental energy to help and often heal the patient, which can deplete their own energy reserves. This is similar to emergency room doctors, nurses, and other healthcare professionals who may find themselves feeling very run down or ill while attempting to treat others.

My understanding is that you can only give out what you yourself have an abundance of. If massage therapists and various other health-related professionals continue to draw from their well (life force, qi, prana) without replenishing it, they will soon face their own health issues. Factors such as exercise, diet, and lifestyle choices all affect the practitioners' own well-being and ability to replenish or maintain their innate life force.

I learned early that you only have so much energy to give. You have to spend it correctly.

Eva Gabor

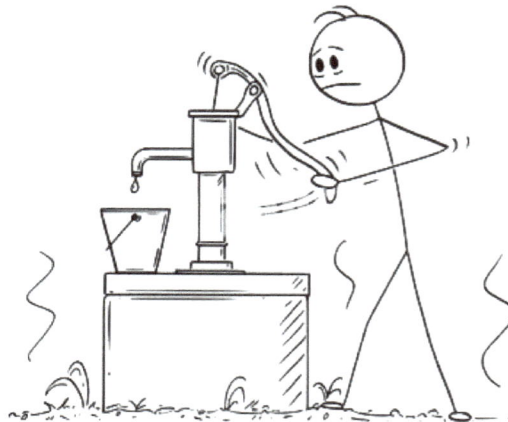

This concept applies to any occupation or activity where one individual loses some level of energy while trying to help another. It includes parents caring for children, caretakers of elderly parents, teachers, and more. It all comes down to the intent behind the actions and the energy expended and received.

This leads to the topic of energy vampires and energy suns. We've likely all encountered people who, upon entering a room, drain the energy of those around them, or conversely, individuals who uplift everyone's energy and bring smiles to everyone's faces. Yin and yang exist in all things!

62

Scarcity vs. Abundance
by Michael Hyatt

SCARCITY	ABUNDANCE
There is never enough	There is always more where that came from
Stingy with knowledge, contacts and compassion	Happy to share knowledge, contacts and compassion
Default to suspicion; hard to build rapport	Default to rapport and build trust easily
Resent competition. Makes the pie smaller, them weaker	Welcome competitors. Makes the pie larger, them stronger
Ask self: How can I get by with less than expected?	Ask self: How can I give more than expected?
Pessimistic about the future; tough times are ahead	Optimistic about the future; the best is yet to come
They think small, avoiding risk	They think big, embracing risk
They are entitled and fearful	They are thankful and confident

SOURCE: http://michaelhyatt.com/064-two-kinds-of-thinkers-podcast.html
Compiled by Chuck Frey, author of *Up Your Impact* - http://upyourimpact.com

Do We Die and Go to Heaven, or Die and Bring Heaven with Us?

Many say they know of the afterlife either being a good place (heaven) or a bad place (hell). Others believe that life here is a temporary classroom, where we keep coming back to revisiting lessons not yet understood. No one alive can truly know the proven existence of any life beyond their current physical manifestation. Some hope for an afterlife that is heavenly but also live a life that is hellish. Quite the quandary, no?

Why not try to live a heavenly life, and hopefully bring that with you when you pass? It sounds better than living in hell on earth and then taking hell with you to the next level of existence. There are many theories regarding the laws of attraction and how we often acquire what we dwell upon, whether deemed as good or bad. Those who think mainly about wealth and/or fame put much of their energy into obtaining these things. However, once they acquire these items, they often realize that they are not truly happy with themselves because they sacrificed things such as family, friends, health, and other aspects of their being.

Others see God's kingdom as heaven on earth. Their life may be full of love, gratitude, and happiness. Some may see their physical life here on earth as hell, with none of the previously mentioned aspects, and therefore look forward to hopefully reaching a better place in the hereafter. The famous philosopher Confucius is thought to have said that we should not focus on the afterlife because we don't understand much about it. Instead, we should focus on our everyday life here in the present.

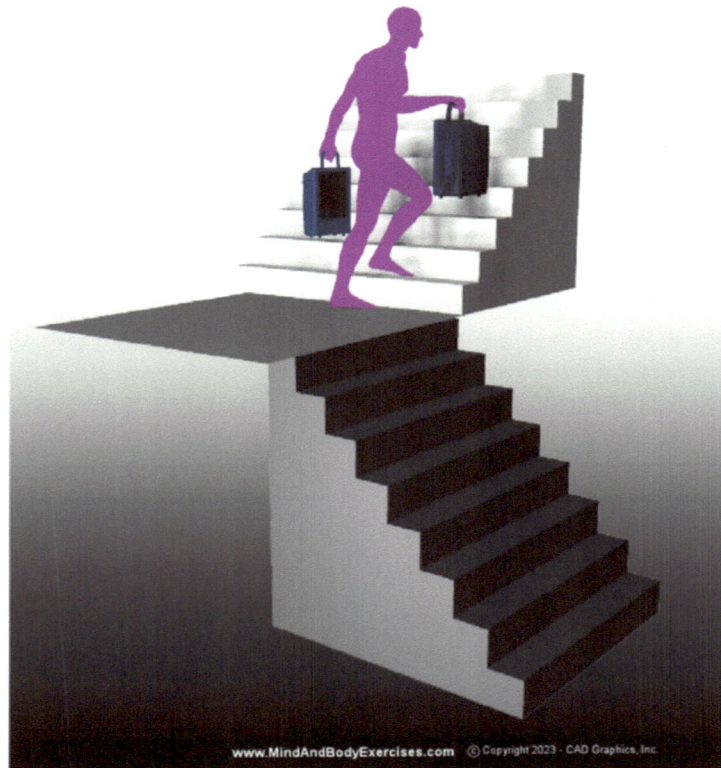

I take this further to mean that we can choose to believe that the Kingdom of God is here right now, in our mind and body, here in the physical world. My understanding is that the state of our thoughts at the very time of our passing is of the utmost importance. What we do or don't do here on Earth within our physical lifetimes can and will affect what happens to our soul or consciousness after our physical being expires.

I have personally been exposed to many people who are most concerned about what may happen in their next life, with very little concern about how they live this current physical life. Others care only about their wants and desires in front of them, with no concerns about what may come next. We may indeed die and go to a place of heaven or hell based upon how we live our lives. If we strive to live a "heavenly-like" life, we may be able to take that peacefulness, joy, and bliss with us to whatever the next phase we have earned. Conversely, if we live a life full of hell in anger, hatred, suffering, and regret, we very well may bring that negative energy to whatever that next place may be.

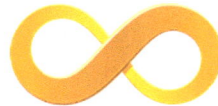

Mastery in the World of Form: Integrating Wealth, Health, and Spirit

In the pursuit of personal evolution, many traditions emphasize the renunciation of material wealth as a path to spiritual enlightenment. Yet this view may overlook an essential truth: the mastery of life requires full engagement with both the spiritual and material realms. Rather than rejecting worldly success, a more holistic path invites individuals to develop discipline, embrace responsibility, and integrate spiritual realization with material abundance.

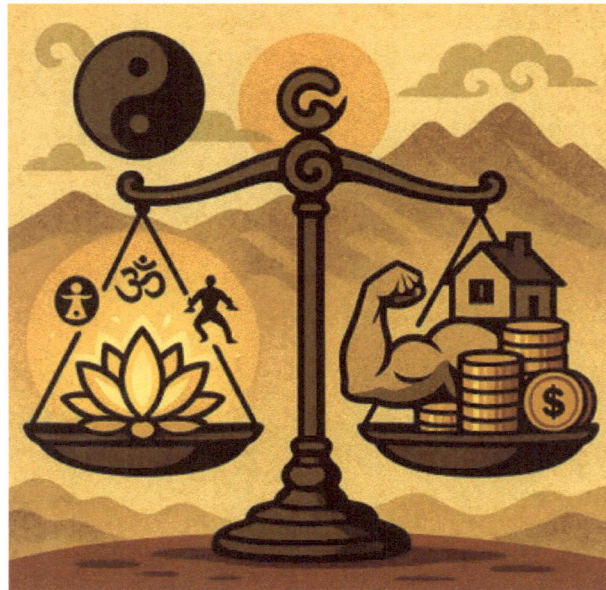

A balanced life requires strength across physical, emotional, and spiritual dimensions. True power, especially in men, is not measured by dominance or accumulation alone, but by maturity and restraint. Without discipline, power can become dangerous, giving rise to instability and harm. Therefore, self-mastery begins with a commitment to personal responsibility, training the body, focusing the mind, and cultivating inner peace.

One foundational concept in this approach is the idea that wealth and health are not opposites of spiritual life but necessary stages in the ladder of awakening. Through conscious acquisition and enjoyment of material pleasures—followed by the ability to release attachment—one gains not only experience but freedom from the cycles of craving and aversion. This path requires mastering the "world of form," learning to participate in it fully without being controlled by it. Those who avoid or bypass this stage may find themselves spiritually incomplete. If one believes in reincarnation, this situation may lead to further experiences in future lifetimes to fully integrate these unlearned lessons.

Conscious development can be mapped through the lens of energy centers or chakras, where each stage corresponds to an essential life lesson: from physical grounding and pleasure to peace, joy, love, compassion, and ultimately ecstatic or blissful states of awareness. These are not mere metaphors but practical tools for tracking one's evolution. A person who cannot access joy or inner peace may need to revisit the foundations of health, safety, and stability before advancing into higher spiritual states.

Seasons of Life - 5 Elements

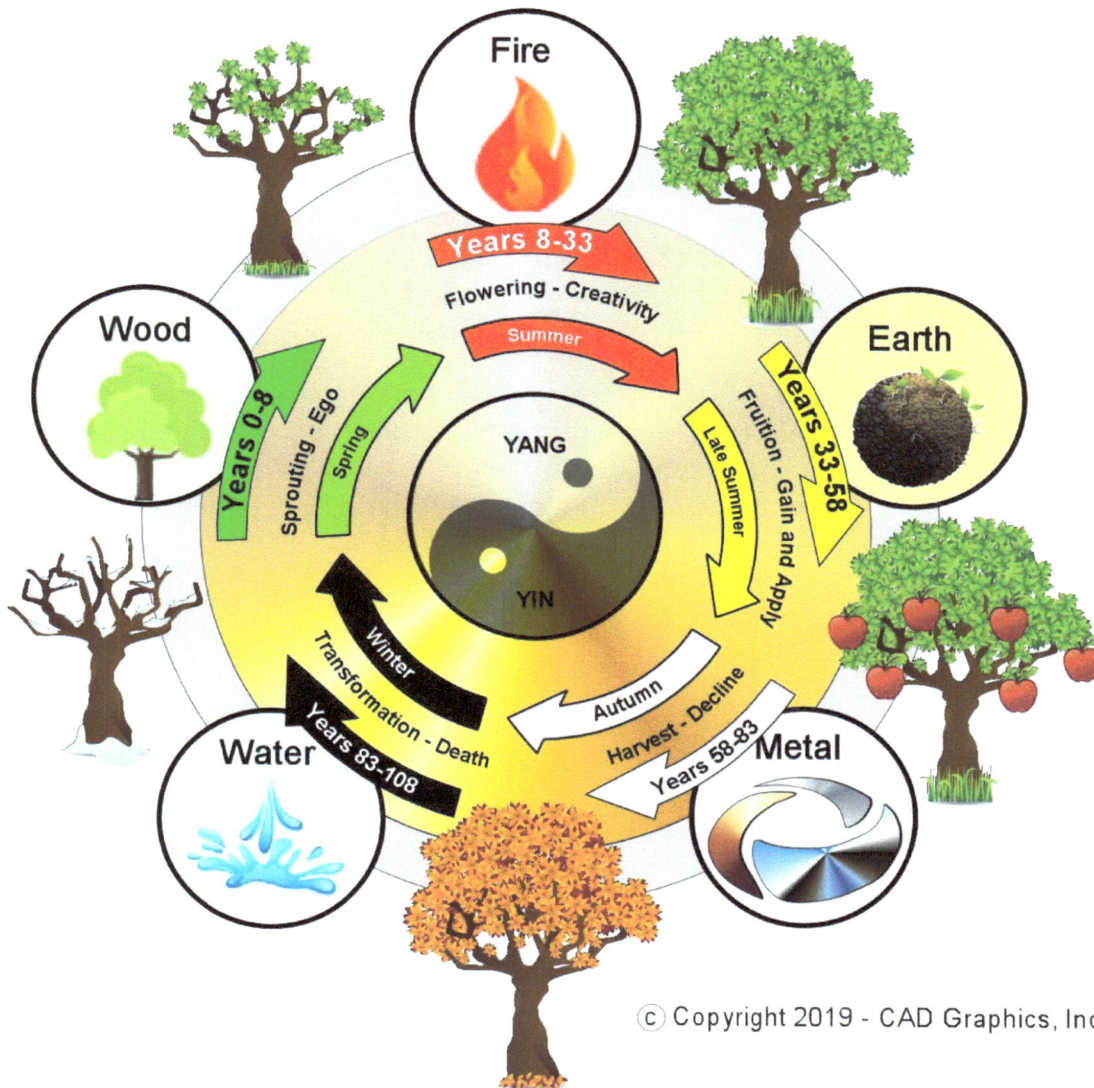

© Copyright 2019 - CAD Graphics, Inc.

Central to this journey is the rejection of victimhood. Blaming society, circumstances, or others for one's failures hinders growth. Only by accepting full responsibility for one's health, finances, relationships, and spiritual development can one initiate true transformation. This principle applies across life stages, which can be seen as cycles: childhood (0–8), adolescence and young adulthood (8–33), fruition (33–58), correction (58–83), and ultimately the sage or spirit phase (83–108). Each phase carries its own lessons and demands appropriate effort and reflection.

In later life, aging should not be viewed as decay, but as a biological and spiritual opportunity. With proper practice through breathwork, meditation, physical cultivation, and mental clarity, many signs of aging can be reversed or mitigated. The aim is to remain vibrant, focused, and spiritually prepared for death, which, when acknowledged consciously, becomes a motivator for authentic living.

The role of family, lineage, and tradition is also pivotal. Respect for one's parents and ancestors does not require blind obedience or emotional entanglement but calls for honoring their place in one's development. This maturity fosters generational healing and sets an example for those who follow.

Integration of spiritual wisdom with material responsibility is not unique to any one culture. Whether through Christian parables, Taoist discipline, or Buddhist insight, timeless truths emerge: the value of discipline, the importance of presence, the need for compassion, and the certainty of death. When viewed through this inclusive lens, spirituality becomes less about belief and more about the embodiment of universal principles.

The ideal individual, a strong, wise, and compassionate being, embodies the archetype of the strategist and warrior. Not through brute strength or spiritual aloofness, but through the unification of effort, enjoyment, reflection, and humility. Mastery is not found in a cave or an office alone, but in the weaving of both. When one lives fully, without excuses or illusions, the path reveals itself not above the world, but through it.

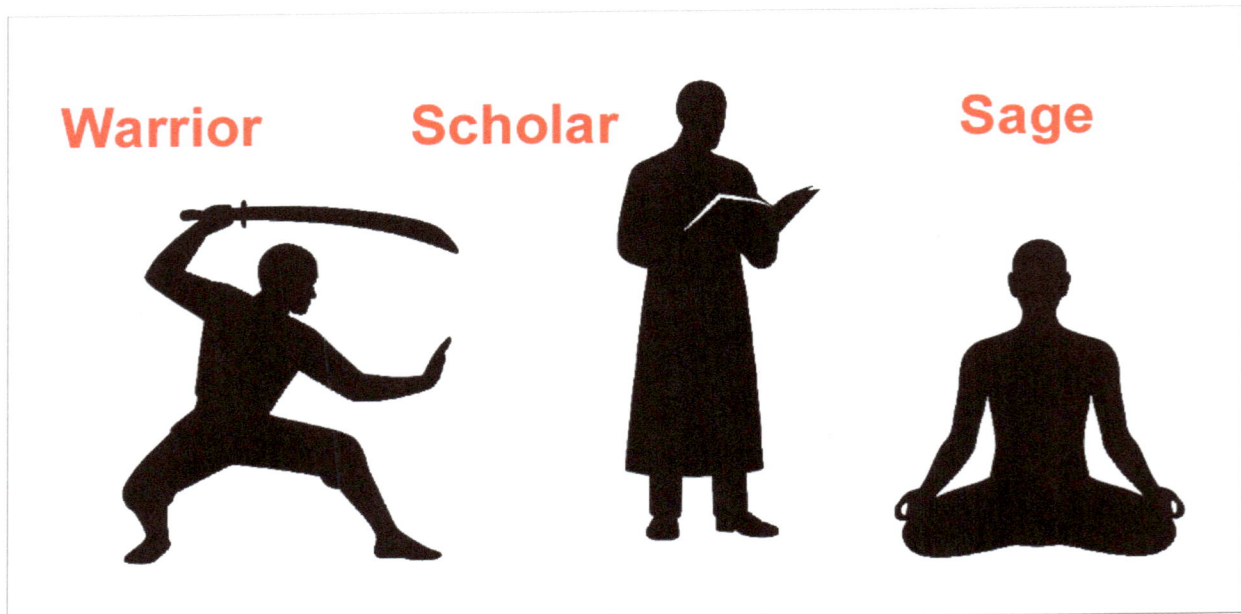

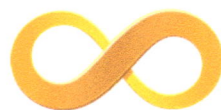

SECTION III: MOVEMENT, TRAINING & PRACTICE METHODS

Bodhidharma's Legacy in Physical and Spiritual Cultivation

The historical narrative of martial arts in China is deeply interwoven with spiritual cultivation, particularly through the legendary influence of **Bodhidharma (Damo)**, the Indian monk credited with introducing *Chan (Zen) Buddhism* to the *Shaolin* Temple. His teachings are widely regarded as the seed of Shaolin martial arts, combining meditative discipline with physical conditioning through systems such as the *YiJin Jing* (Muscle-Tendon Changing Classic) and the *18 Luohan Hands*. These practices, over centuries, evolved into the sophisticated combat and wellness system now known as Shaolin Kung Fu.

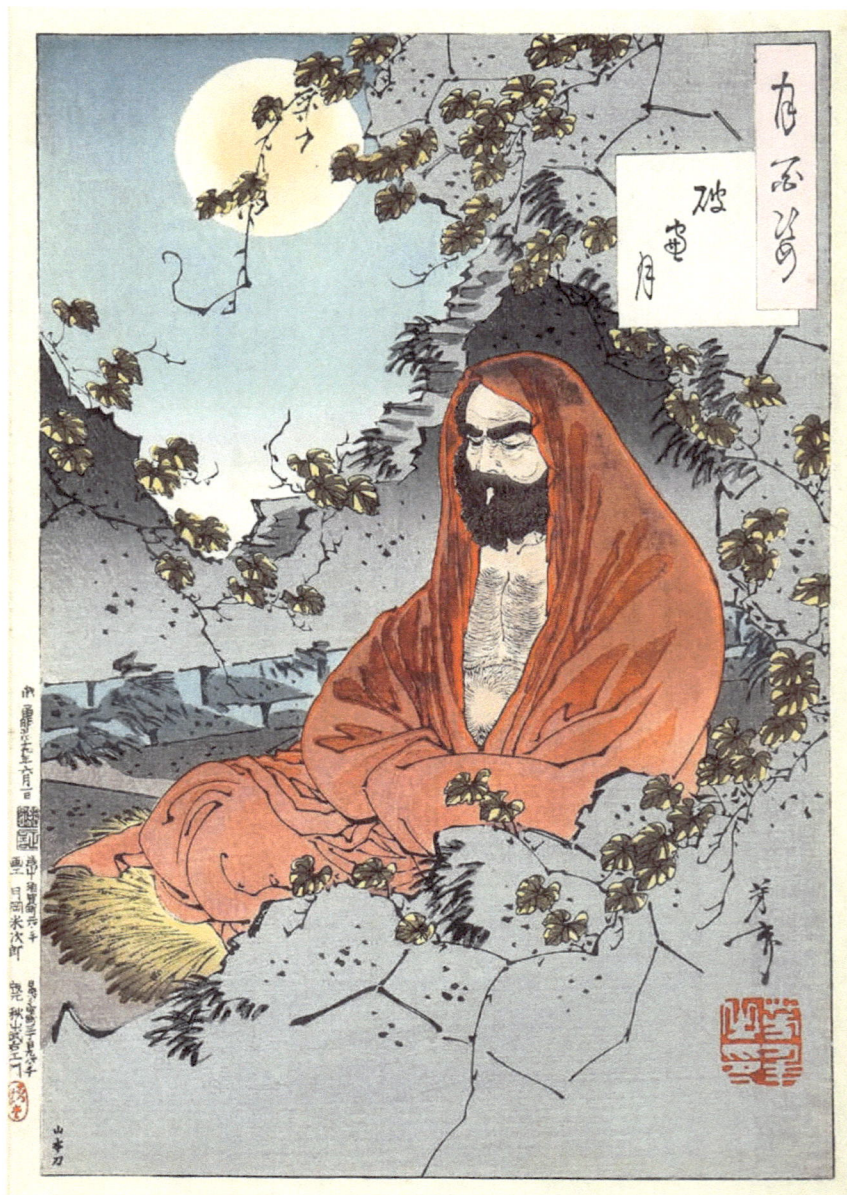

Bodhidharma's Contributions

Bodhidharma's arrival at the Shaolin Monastery in roughly the 5th or 6th century CE introduced transformative practices focused on both internal and external cultivation. He is traditionally credited with teaching three major systems:

Chan meditation - promoted inner stillness and enlightenment through direct experience and introspection (Red Pine, 1987)

YiJin Jing (Muscle and Tendon Changing) and *Xisui Jing* (Marrow Cleansing Classic). Which the two were physical regimens aimed at strengthening the body, improving Qi circulation, and preparing monks for long periods of seated meditation (Shahar, 2008).

YiJin Jing: Conditioning the Body for Higher Purpose

The *YiJin Jing* consists of dynamic tension exercises that train the musculature, tendons, and fascia, preparing the body not only for martial use but also for maintaining vitality and structural integrity. These exercises, according to tradition, were prescribed by Bodhidharma to enhance the monks' endurance and resistance to fatigue and essential for rigorous spiritual practices (Henning, 1999). Movements from YiJin *Jing* later evolved into practical combat sequences, emphasizing controlled breathing, rooted stances, and explosive force, characteristics now central to Shaolin martial arts.

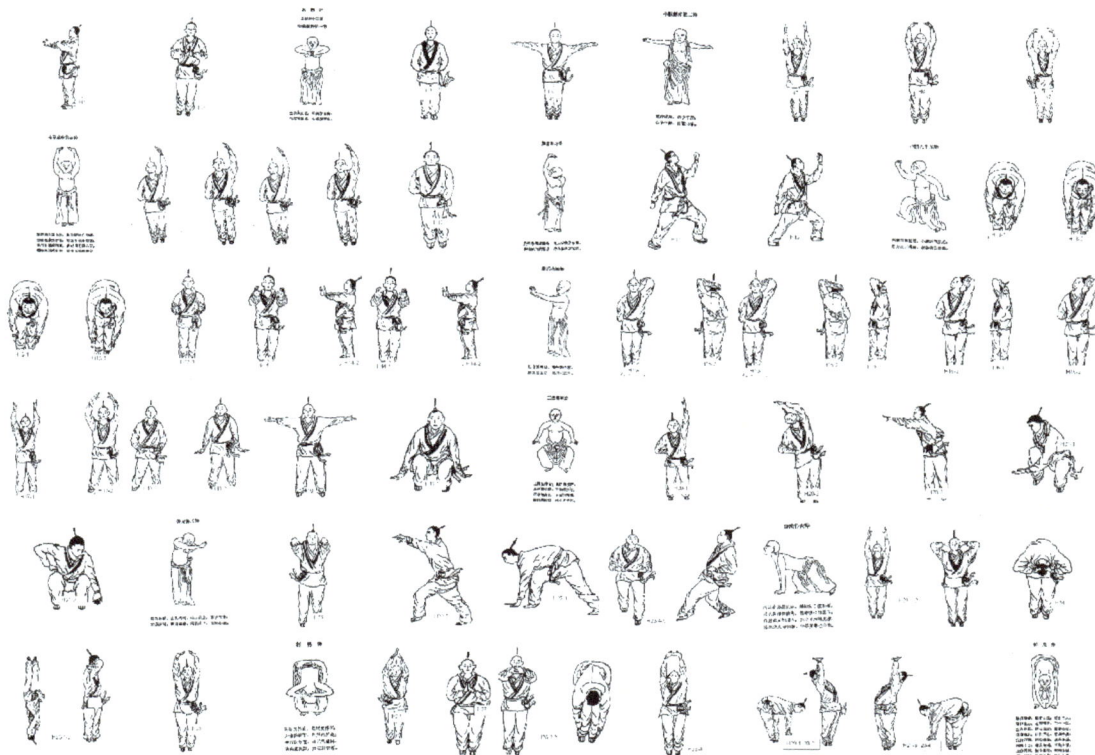

http://blogtiengviet.net/NghiaHa

YiJin Jing (Muscle & Tendon Changing)

18 Luohan Hands: The Proto-Forms of Shaolin Kung Fu

The *18 Luohan Hands* are a set of Qigong-like movements, traditionally considered the earliest structured exercises linking health cultivation and martial efficacy. These forms included basic palm strikes, circular motions, and integrated breath control. These elements would later become foundational for Shaolin fighting systems. Over time, they were elaborated into more complex forms such as *Luohanquan* (Arhat Fist), a style known for its precise, direct strikes and meditative underpinnings (Shahar, 2008).

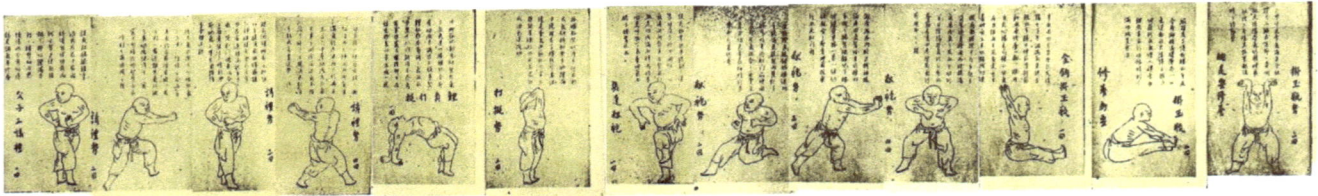

13 Luohan Qigong: Bridging Internal and External

A related tradition, *13 Luohan Qigong*, comprises a sequence of exercises that further integrates internal energy development with martial readiness. Each of the 13 movements targets specific energetic pathways and anatomical functions. For instance, "Luohan Draws the Bow" emphasizes lung expansion and Qi projection, while "Luohan Stands on One Leg" cultivates balance and stability. These movements not only reinforce martial mechanics but also nurture internal harmony, resonating with Taoist and Buddhist philosophies on health and enlightenment (Yang, 2010).

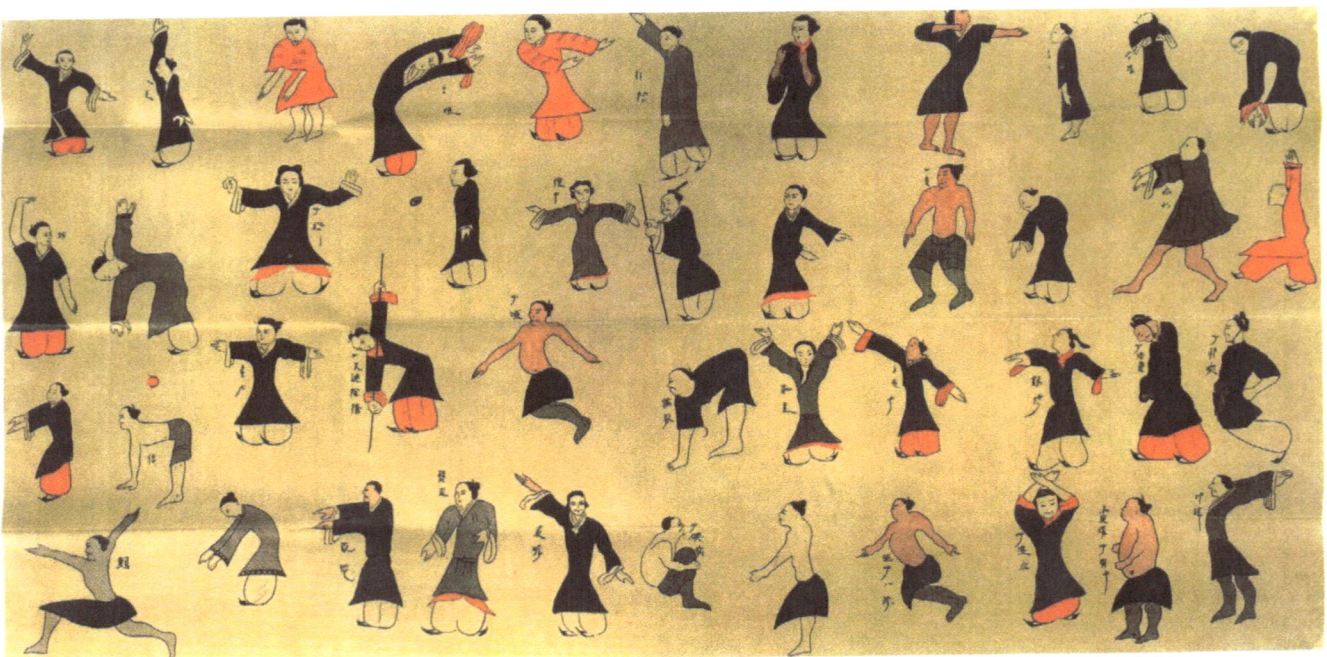

The Synthesis into Shaolin Martial Arts

The transition from static Qigong forms to combative martial art forms at Shaolin was catalyzed by the necessity of self-defense and discipline. The YiJin Jing provided the physiological robustness and tendon strength required for explosive movement, while the *18 Luohan Hands* offered the basic motor patterns and coordination that could be adapted into fighting techniques. By combining these with Chan Buddhist principles and eventually incorporating external influences such as Chinese military tactics and folk styles, Shaolin monks developed a comprehensive martial system.

This system expanded into various forms and weapons styles, each integrating internal power (*Nei Dan*), structural integrity, and mental discipline. Notably, *Luohanquan* emerged as a canonical representation of these origins, continuing the legacy of the original Luohan exercises through its focus on both spirit and technique (Wong, 1996).

Conclusion

The legacy of Bodhidharma at Shaolin Temple is not only spiritual but deeply physical. Through systems such as YiJin Jing, 18 Luohan Hands, and 13 Luohan Qigong, he set in motion a lineage that would unite body, mind, and spirit into one of the world's most enduring martial traditions. Today, practitioners of Shaolin arts continue to embody these principles, integrating ancient wisdom with modern discipline in the pursuit of balance, strength, and self-realization.

References:

Henning, S. E. (1999). Academia encounters the Chinese martial arts. *China Review International*, 6(2), 319–332. https://www.jstor.org/stable/23732172

Pine, R. (1987). THE ZEN TEACHING of Bodhidharma. In *North Point Press* (First). North Point Press. https://selfdefinition.org/zen/Zen-Teaching-of-Bodhidharma-trans-Red-Pine-clearscan.pdf

Shahar, M. (2008). *The Shaolin Monastery: History, Religion, and the Chinese Martial Arts*. University of Hawai'i Press. *www.jstor.org*. https://www.jstor.org/stable/j.ctvvmxs5

Wong, Kiew Kit. (1996). *The Art of Shaolin Kung Fu: The Secrets of Kung Fu for Self-Defense, Health, and Enlightenment*. Tuttle Publishing.

Yang, Jwing-Ming. (2010). *Qigong Meditation: Embryonic Breathing*. YMAA Publication Center. https://ymaa.com/articles/qigong-meditation/embryonic-breathing

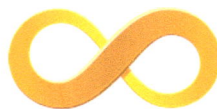

Wind and Water, Makes Fire

The human mind and body are integral parts of nature, constantly interacting with its energies. There is a direct correlation between the systems of nature and those of the body, with three key elements of wind, fire, and water, serving as points of connection.

-   **Wind** corresponds to the respiratory system, as the air we breathe sustains life.

-   **Fire** represents body temperature, which plays a vital role in all physiological functions.

-   **Water** relates to the circulatory system, essential for vitality and well-being.

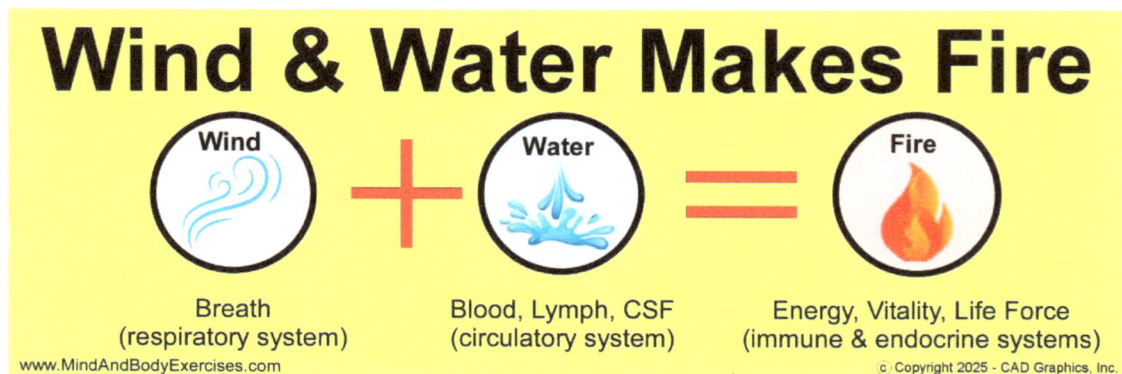

Wind & Water Makes Fire

Wind + Water = Fire

Breath
(respiratory system)

Blood, Lymph, CSF
(circulatory system)

Energy, Vitality, Life Force
(immune & endocrine systems)

www.MindAndBodyExercises.com   © Copyright 2025 - CAD Graphics, Inc.

Practices such as Tai Chi, Qigong, and Bagua Zhang profoundly influence the body, impacting the organs, joints, and muscles at a deep level. In Taoist alchemy, the philosophical phrase **_"wind and water make fire"_** metaphorically represents the dynamic interactions of the Five Elements (Wu Xing) and the internal processes of self-cultivation.

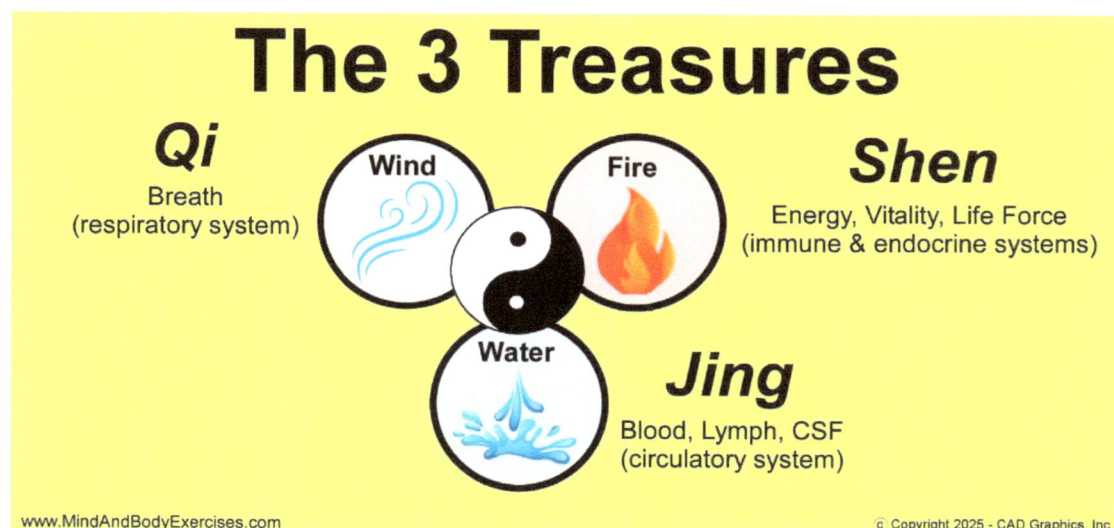

The 3 Treasures

Qi
Breath
(respiratory system)

Wind

Fire

Shen
Energy, Vitality, Life Force
(immune & endocrine systems)

Water

Jing
Blood, Lymph, CSF
(circulatory system)

www.MindAndBodyExercises.com   © Copyright 2025 CAD Graphics, Inc.

Here's a breakdown of how this concept fits into Taoist thought:

Five Elements Correspondence:
- **Wind (Feng, 风)** is often associated with Wood (Mu, 木), which represents growth, movement, and expansion.

- **Water (Shui, 水)** corresponds to the Kidneys and the essence (Jing), which serves as the foundation for transformation.

- **Fire (Huo, 火)** corresponds to Yang energy, warmth, and spirit (Shen).

- The idea is that the interaction of movement (Wind/Wood) and nourishment (Water) can generate Fire (Yang energy, transformation).

Neidan (Internal Alchemy) Interpretation:
- Wind (Wood) and Water represent Qi and Jing, respectively.

- Their controlled interaction through breathwork, meditation, and energy circulation can generate the internal *"alchemy fire"* needed to refine essence into Qi and Qi into Shen.

- This fire is not literal but the internal warmth and energetic transformation that happens in deep meditation or Qigong.

Martial & Qigong Perspective:
- In advanced Qigong and martial arts, regulated breath (Wind) and internal fluid movement (Water) manifest into internal heat (Fire), leading to refined power and vitality.

- This aligns with practices of Tai Chi, Qigong and BaguaZhang, where breath, body movement, and mind-intent cultivate the internal fire for vitality and martial efficiency.

Wind & Water Makes Fire

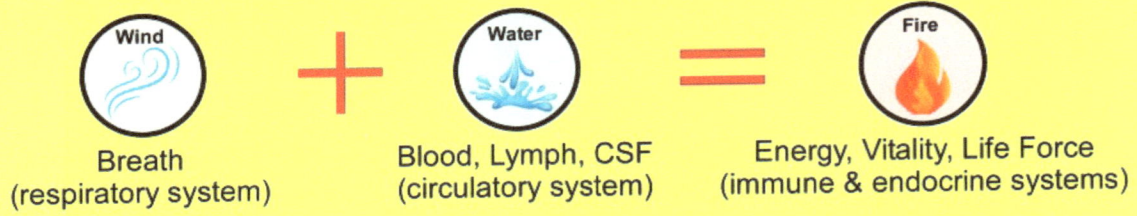

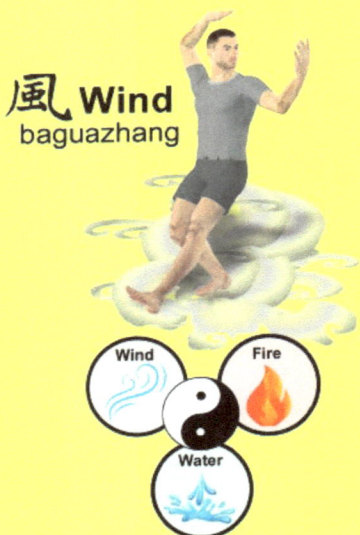

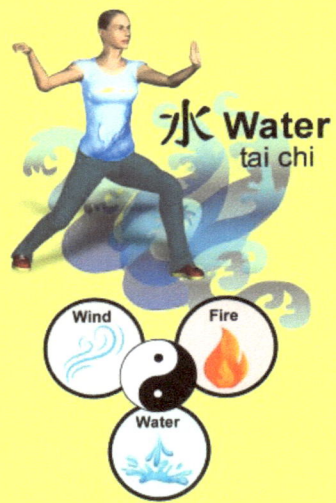

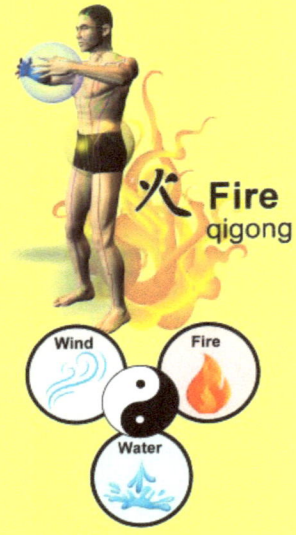

Wind + **Water** = **Fire**

Breath
(respiratory system)

Blood, Lymph, CSF
(circulatory system)

Energy, Vitality, Life Force
(immune & endocrine systems)

風 **Wind**
baguazhang

水 **Water**
tai chi

火 **Fire**
qigong

each practice has components of wind, water & fire

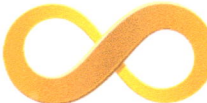

Before there was Crossfit, there was isometric, aerobic and anaerobic training. Before there was functional training, martial arts utilized exercises that were performance as well as fitness and wellness. Before organized martial arts, there was qigong and its parent of yoga, where exercises were focused on achieving a balanced relationship between the mind, body and self-awareness (spiritual). Many modern exercise and wellness concepts, draw from ancient knowledge and understanding of how humans coexist within nature and not separate from it.

Good health of the lower back starts with good posture. The following set of exercises develop strength, increase muscular range of motion and to a lesser degree – flexibility. Strength in the back, hips and abdomen, provide a strong cage that houses the internal organs. Flexibility in these areas helps to maintain good blood circulation to the organs and lower body. Unique to this set of exercises is the body postures combined with holding a weighted object and the extra awareness required to hold it while also maintaining the correct body alignments. By holding the bottle at the top using only the fingertips, the nervous system is engaged throughout the whole body. Try to hold the static positions or perform moving exercises from 20 seconds to longer intervals such as 1, 2, 5 minutes or longer, to achieve advanced levels of development physically and mentally. Holding positions generally develops strength whereas repetitive movements develop flexibility and endurance. Relax the body into the positions in spite of any tension in the muscles. Deep and relaxed breathing is essential while performing these exercises.

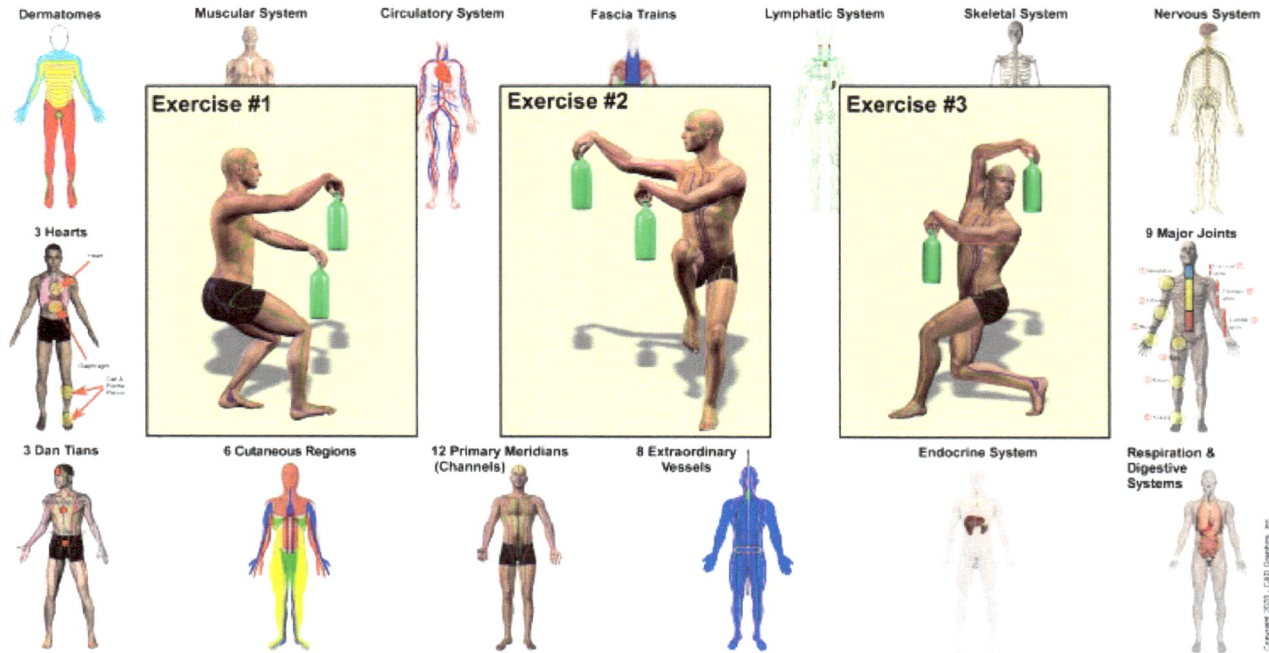

Advanced levels of physical and mental strength can be achieved by holding these positions for longer periods of time. Start slowly by holding on one side for a few seconds and then switching to the opposite side. Your determination will increase by trying to hold the bottles up without allowing them to drop from your fingertips. Also, holding the postures longer without failure will dramatically increase mental strength and tolerance to pain and stress.

After diligent practice, over a few months of continuous training, 1-5 minutes can be an obtainable amount of time to hold the bottles and body positions without taking a break from switching to the opposite side. Another variation of these exercises would be to adjust the amount of weight or water in the bottles. Begin with a nearly empty 16-ounce bottle. Eventually, add more water working up to a 2-liter soda bottle over a few months' time.

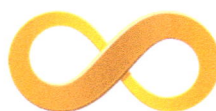

Shim Yuk – A practice to engage the mind and body

Health and fitness enthusiasts often are in search of the next best fitness gadget to take them to the next challenge or maybe just increase variety in their routine. For hundreds of years and probably more, martial arts have offered a wide spectrum of what is today marketed as flow-yoga, Cross Fit, function training, high intensity training (HIT) and others. Using simple apparatus that can be obtained from Home Depot, or other retailers can offer unlimited options to achieve whatever fitness levels are desired, without ridiculous membership fees or equipment costs. An example of how our culture still thinks that we can buy our way to wellness, is paying $1500-$3000 for a stationary exercise bike when $50 worth of odds and ends can do the job (and often better). Either way, YOU have to do the work to achieve YOUR fitness, wellness and relative happiness.

Shim Yuk - Whole Body Engagement

The nervous system innervates the muscles that are engaged during practice of the Shim Yuk exercises. Additionally, the cardiopulmonary and skeletal systems are also engaged. Focused thought is necessary in order to maintain the correct posture while executing each repetition.

Cervical Muscles:
sternocleidomastoid
scalenus
spinalis cervicis
spinalis capitus
semispinalis cervicis
semispinalis capitus
splenius cervicis
longus colli cervicis
longus capitus

rectus capitus anterior
rectus capitus lateralis
Iliocostalis cervicis
longissimus cervicis
longissimus capitis
rectus capitus posterior major
rectus capitus posterior minor
obliquus capitus Inferior
obliquus capitus superior

Thoracic Muscles:
longissimus thoracis
Iliocostalis thoracis
spinalis thoracis
semispinalis thoracis
rotatores thoracis

Muscles of the Buttocks:
gluteus maximus
gluteus medius
gluteus minimus

Quadricep Muscles:
rectus femoris
vastus lateralis
vastus intermedius
vastus medialis

Lumbar Muscles:
psoas major
Intertransversarii lateralis
quadratus lumborum
Interspinales
Intertransversarii mediales
multifidus
longissimus lumborum
Iliocostalis lumborum

Hamstring Muscle Group:
semitendinosus
semimembranosus
biceps femoris

ankle muscles:
gastrocnemius
soleus
tibialis posterior
tibialis anterior
peroneus longus
peroneus brevis
flexor hallucis longus
flexor digitorum longus
extensor hallucis longus
extensor digitorum longus

Shoulder, Arm & Chest Muscles:
infraspinatus
triceps brachii
pectoralis major
pectoralis minor
teres major
biceps brachii
latissimus dorsi
subscapularis
supraspinatus

Hand & Wrist Muscles:
abductor digiti minimi
abductor pollicis brevis
abductor pollicis longus
adductor pollicis
brachioradialis
dorsal expansion (hood)
dorsal Interosseous
extensor carpi radialis brevis
extensor carpi radialis longus
extensor carpi ulnaris
extensor digiti minimi
extensor digitorum
extensor Indicis
extensor pollicis brevis
extensor retinaculum
flexor carpi radialis
flexor carpi ulnaris
flexor digiti minimi brevis
flexor digitorum profundus
flexor digitorum superficialis
flexor pollicis brevis
flexor retinaculum
lumbrical muscles
opponens pollicis
palmar Interosseous
palmaris longus
pronator quadratus

Muscles of the Foot:
flexor hallucis brevis
abductor hallucis
flexor digitorum longus
lumbricals
flexor digitorum brevis
quadratus plantae

www.MindAndBodyExercises.com

© copyright 2022 · CAD Graphics, Inc.

Unique to this exercise called "Shim Yuk", is the body posture combined with holding a weighted object and the extra awareness required to hold it stable while also maintaining the correct body alignments. By holding the pole level, moving only the hands and wrists, the fascia trains, the nervous, muscular and skeletal systems are all engaged throughout the entire body. Theories abound regarding the activation of our inherit ability to heal our own illnesses, also known as "vis medicatrix". Exercises like this, engage our mind, body and spirit thereby, helping to engage "the healing power of nature".

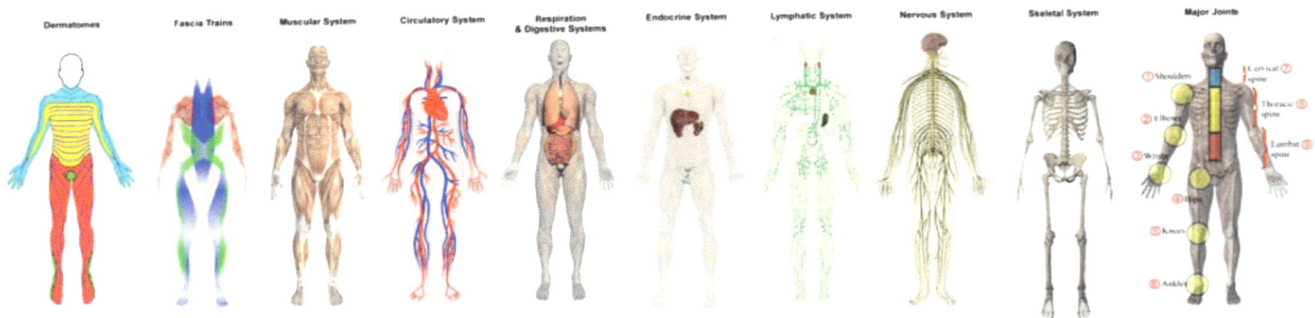

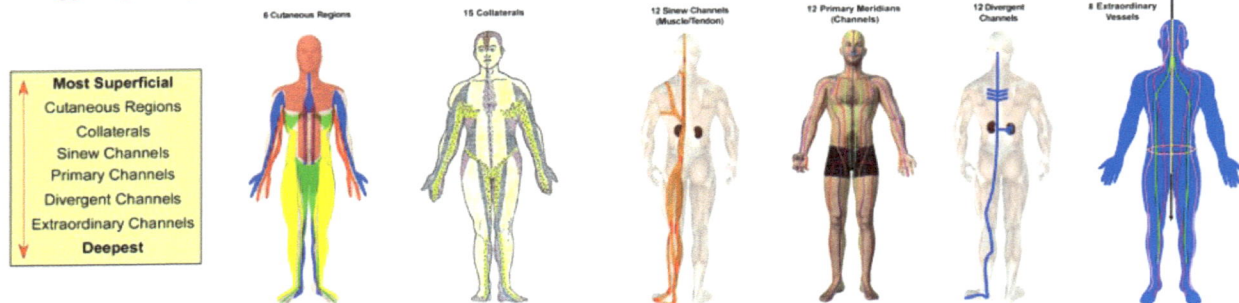

Developing a strong grip is directly related to preventing falls.

The strength of one's grip when they begin to lose their balance, can be the difference between free-falling to the ground and potential bone fracture, or catching one's balance by grabbing a rail or other stationary structure. Shim Yuk practice definitely goes way beyond being just a hand/wrist strengthening exercise. However, this exercise will produce phenomenal hand and wrist strength if practiced diligently.

Try to hold the static position while performing the wrist exercise, from 1, 2, 3, etc. consecutive repetitions. Holding the stance generally develops overall strength whereas repetitive rolling develops stamina, endurance and determination. Relax the body into the positions in spite of any tension in the muscles. Deep and relaxed breathing is essential while performing this exercise.

From my experience of over 40 years of martial arts, fitness and wellness training and teaching, I have seen some amazing benefits coming from shim yuk practice. For those in fairly good shape, one can develop an amazing amount of strength in the wrists, forearms, shoulders, lower back and legs. I have also trained individuals that have had more serious issues such as cerebral palsy, knee injuries, severe trauma to the spine and hip and other ailments that have shown great improvement.

Wrist and Hand Anatomy

Deeper Palmar up Dissection of Right Hand

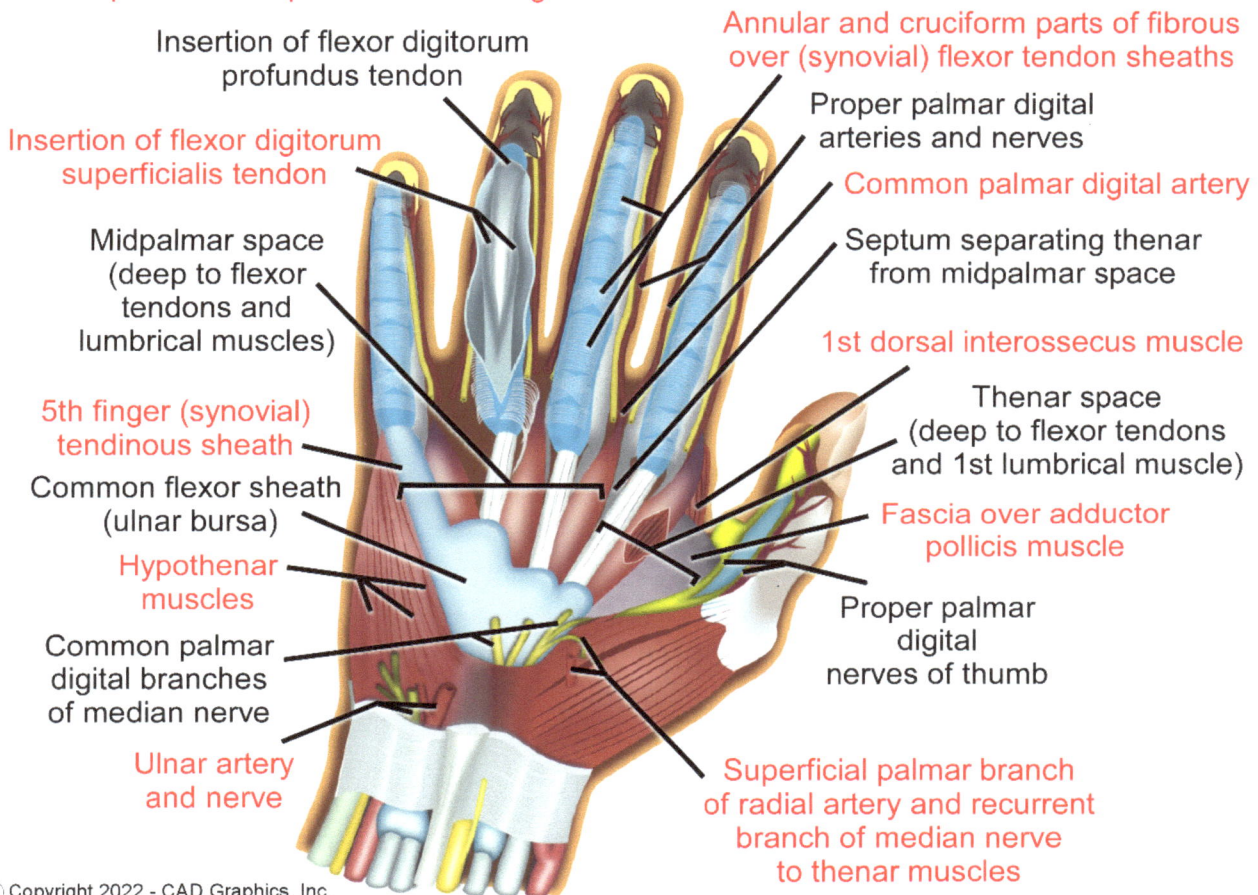

Insertion of flexor digitorum profundus tendon

Insertion of flexor digitorum superficialis tendon

Midpalmar space (deep to flexor tendons and lumbrical muscles)

5th finger (synovial) tendinous sheath

Common flexor sheath (ulnar bursa)

Hypothenar muscles

Common palmar digital branches of median nerve

Ulnar artery and nerve

Annular and cruciform parts of fibrous over (synovial) flexor tendon sheaths

Proper palmar digital arteries and nerves

Common palmar digital artery

Septum separating thenar from midpalmar space

1st dorsal interossecus muscle

Thenar space (deep to flexor tendons and 1st lumbrical muscle)

Fascia over adductor pollicis muscle

Proper palmar digital nerves of thumb

Superficial palmar branch of radial artery and recurrent branch of median nerve to thenar muscles

Strong bones prevent fractures from falling, osteopenia and osteoporosis

Shim Yuk practice strengthens muscles which consequently strengthens bones, which helps to prevent osteopenia (bone loss) and osteoporosis (severe bone density loss). Wolff's Law states that bones become stronger and thicker over time to resist forces placed upon them and weaker and thinner if there are no forces to act against. This principle is important for preventing injuries. Thicker bones are harder to break.

Wolff's Law

Wolff's Law states that our bones become thicker and stronger over time to resist forces placed upon them and thinner and weaker if there are no forces to act against. Wolff's Law and Injury. This principle is important for preventing injuries. A thicker bone is harder to break.

Tension and compression cycles create a small electrical potential that stimulates bone deposition and increased density at points of stress.

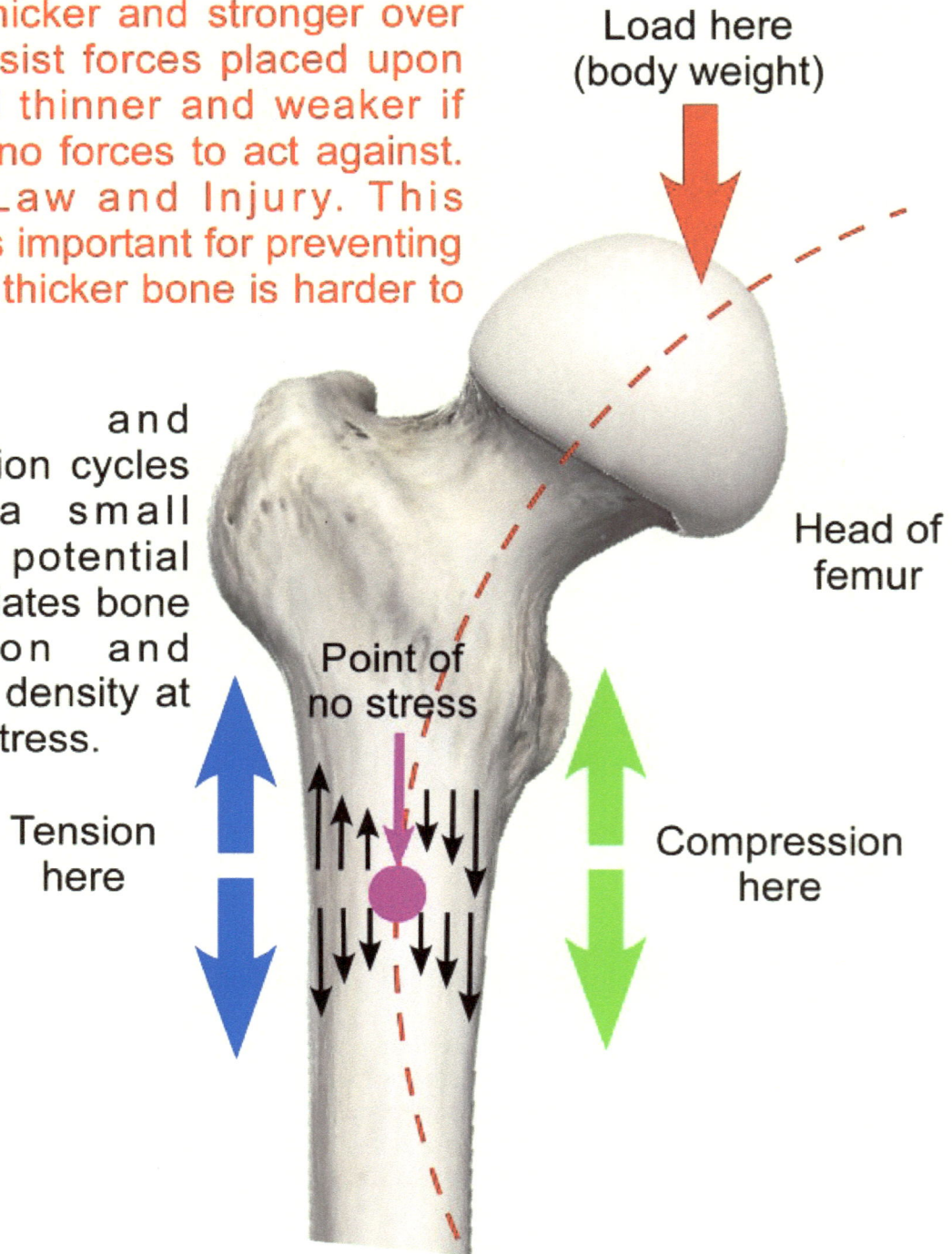

Load here
(body weight)

Head of femur

Point of no stress

Tension here

Compression here

Learning from information on the internet, from video or books can be good. However, to truly get proper instruction, in-person training is usually the best method. Contact me if you have a desire to learn these methods correctly.

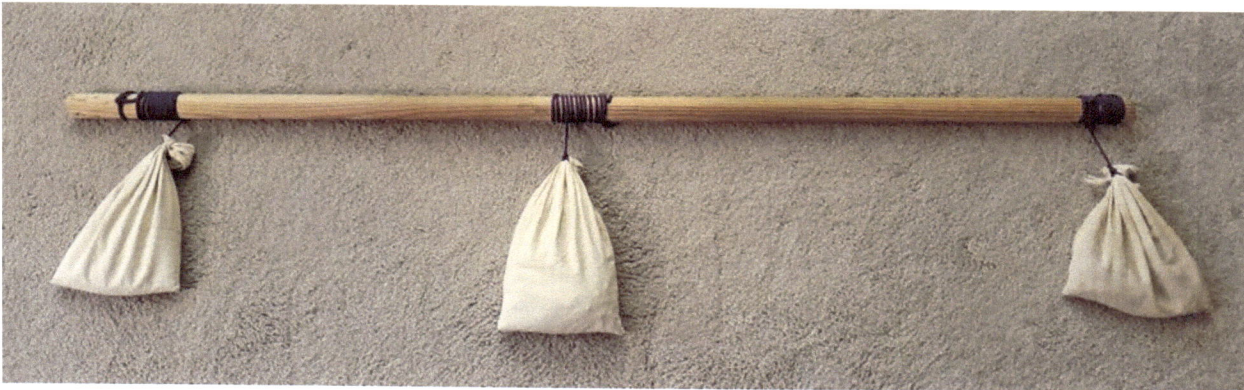

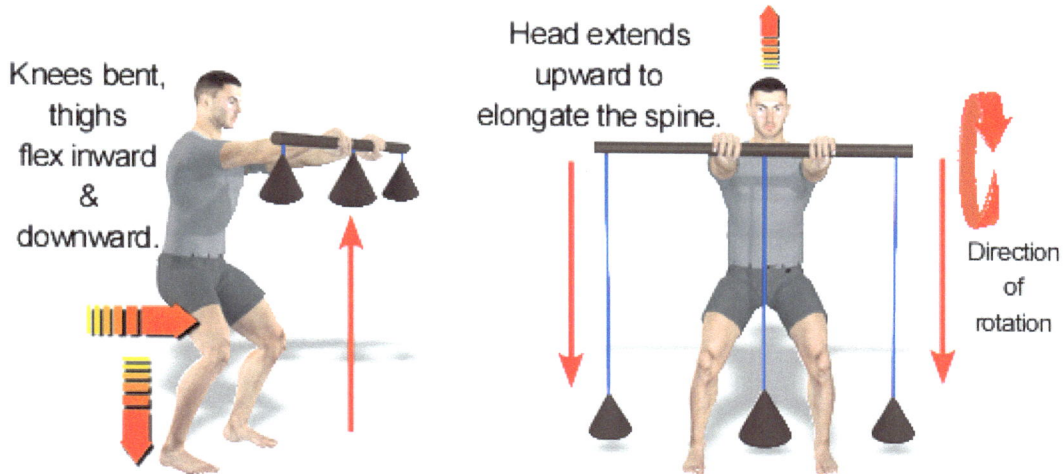

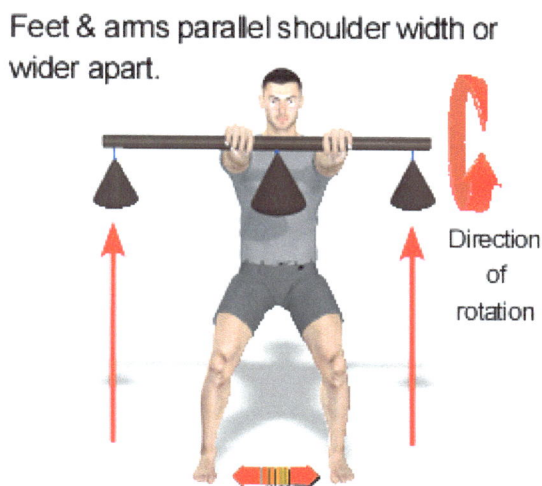

Knees bent, thighs flex inward & downward.

Head extends upward to elongate the spine.

Direction of rotation

Feet & arms parallel shoulder width or wider apart.

Direction of rotation

Just like the tensegrity model, tension on one area of the body can affect tension on all components throughout the human body.

SECTION IV: TRADITIONAL MEDICINE & BODY FUNCTION

Address the Root Causes of Pain and Illness

Allopathic, biomedicine or Western medicine are based upon treating illness through pharmaceuticals, surgery, and other invasive treatments. This approach works well for traumatic injuries and some life-threatening diseases but often falls quite short in treating chronic illnesses due to choices in diet and lifestyle. Allopathic medicine basically puts the healthcare provider in the role of maintaining the health of the individual instead of the individual being responsible for the consequences of their own actions, whether deemed as good or bad for that individual. This is one of the main reasons why healthcare in the US is so expensive, while at the same time our standard of health and wellness rates are far below the best when compared to other countries in the world.

The US does not really provide healthcare but rather encourages "sick care" over self-care.

Find and research the root cause of your disease, pain or discomfort to help become empowered to make your own educated decisions that affect your health and well-being. It is often very difficult to live a comfortable life, when someone has so much pain and suffering within it. The keys to happiness are truly in our own hands.

Self-discipline is the master key to do what we know needs to be done:

– maintain a nutritional diet

– consistently exercise and/or be active

– prioritize sleep quality- nurture healthy social interactions

– get fresh air and some sunlight everyday

– be more positive than negative in your outlook and input

Naturopathic medicine does a fantastic job of outlining how to maintain health and well-being, without 1st jumping to pharmaceutical, surgery and other invasive treatments, before accessing what is appropriate and best for the individual and their particular circumstances. Other medical modalities such as chiropractic and Traditional Chinese Medicine often follow these same principles.

Address the Root Causes of Pain and Illness

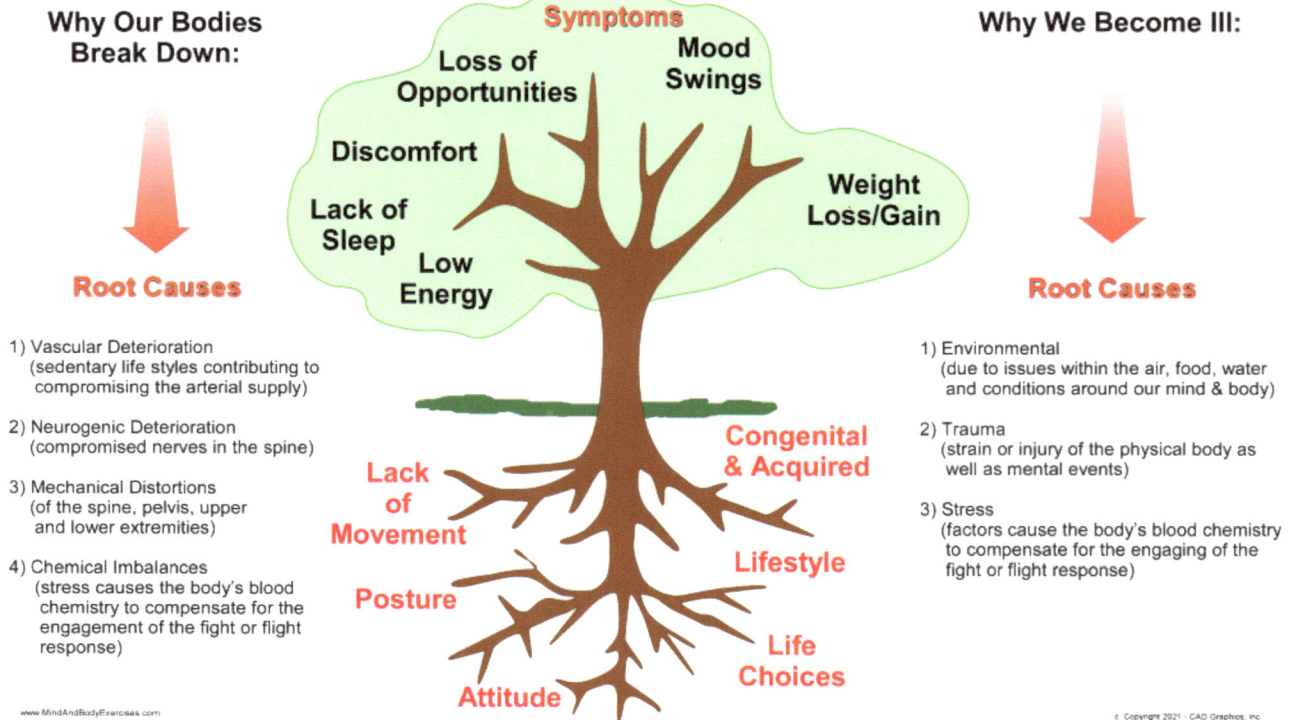

Why Our Bodies Break Down:

Symptoms

- Loss of Opportunities
- Mood Swings
- Discomfort
- Weight Loss/Gain
- Lack of Sleep
- Low Energy

Why We Become Ill:

Root Causes

1) Vascular Deterioration (sedentary life styles contributing to compromising the arterial supply)

2) Neurogenic Deterioration (compromised nerves in the spine)

3) Mechanical Distortions (of the spine, pelvis, upper and lower extremities)

4) Chemical Imbalances (stress causes the body's blood chemistry to compensate for the engagement of the fight or flight response)

Root Causes

1) Environmental (due to issues within the air, food, water and conditions around our mind & body)

2) Trauma (strain or injury of the physical body as well as mental events)

3) Stress (factors cause the body's blood chemistry to compensate for the engaging of the fight or flight response)

- Lack of Movement
- Congenital & Acquired
- Posture
- Lifestyle
- Attitude
- Life Choices

www.MindAndBodyExercises.com

© Copyright 2021 - CAD Graphics, Inc

The Seven-Level Naturopathic

1 - Establish the Conditions for Health

2 - Stimulate the Vis Medicatrix Naturae and Self-Healing Processes

3 - Support and Balance Physiologic and Bioenergetic Systems

4 - Address or Correct Structural Integrity

5 - Address Pathology using Specific Natural Substances or Interventions

6 - Address Pathology using Pharmaceutical or Synthetic Substances

7 - Suppress or Surgically Remove Pathology

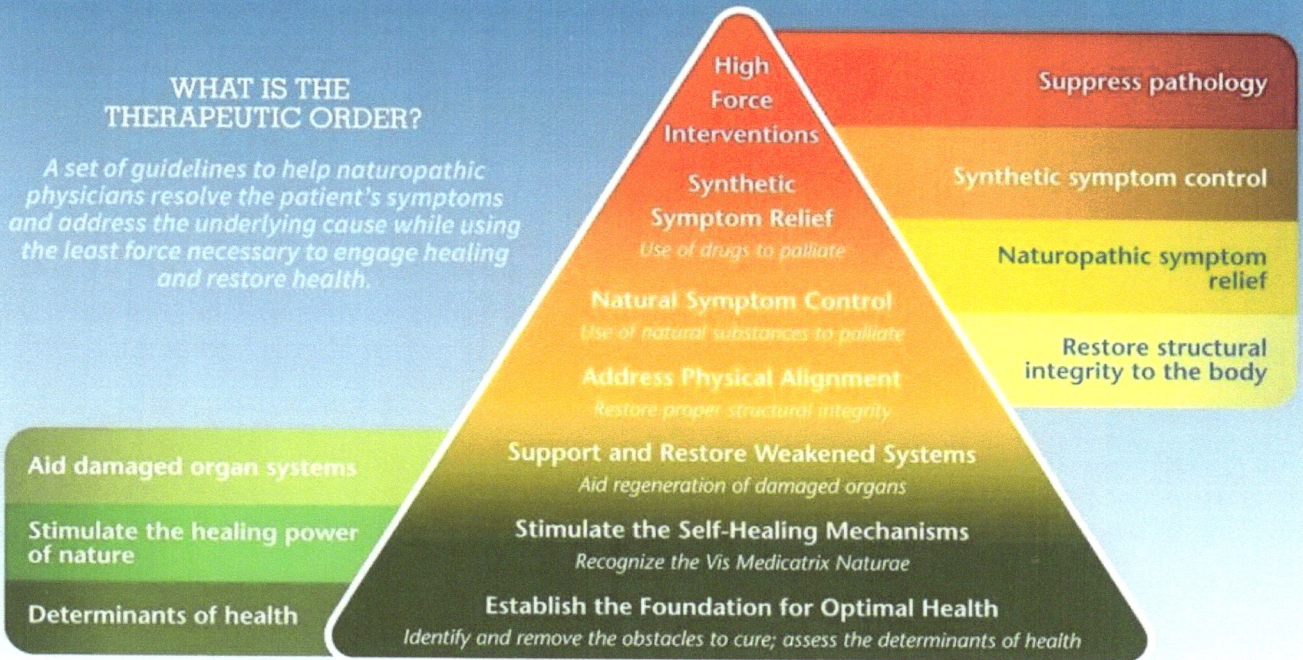

THE THERAPEUTIC ORDER

WHAT IS THE THERAPEUTIC ORDER?

A set of guidelines to help naturopathic physicians resolve the patient's symptoms and address the underlying cause while using the least force necessary to engage healing and restore health.

High Force Interventions — Suppress pathology

Synthetic Symptom Relief — *Use of drugs to palliate* — Synthetic symptom control

Natural Symptom Control — *Use of natural substances to palliate* — Naturopathic symptom relief

Address Physical Alignment — *Restore proper structural integrity* — Restore structural integrity to the body

Support and Restore Weakened Systems — *Aid regeneration of damaged organs*

Stimulate the Self-Healing Mechanisms — *Recognize the Vis Medicatrix Naturae*

Establish the Foundation for Optimal Health — *Identify and remove the obstacles to cure; assess the determinants of health*

Aid damaged organ systems

Stimulate the healing power of nature

Determinants of health

www.fnminstitute.org

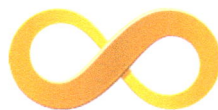

If not having disease or illness is our goal, we need to focus on being fit, well & healthy. Good health usually comes at a cost of time, effort, sacrifice and resources, or a combination of the prior. Most people don't care to make the investment into taking care of themselves until after they are injured. Even then, most people with health issues often choose pain medicines or sometimes surgery over exercise or lifestyle changes that can improve their situation. Traumatic injuries are often best treated with emergency surgery and that is really not the topic of this post.

What is kinetic linking?

The kinetic link principle describes how the human body can be considered in terms of a series of interrelated links or segments. Movement of one segment affects segments both proximal and distal to the first segment.

Like a machine, it's made up of otherwise fixed segments given mobility by joints. A kinetic chain is the notion that these joints and segments have an effect on one another during movement. When one is in motion, it creates a chain of events that affect the movement of neighboring joints and segments.

"When one-part moves, all parts move"

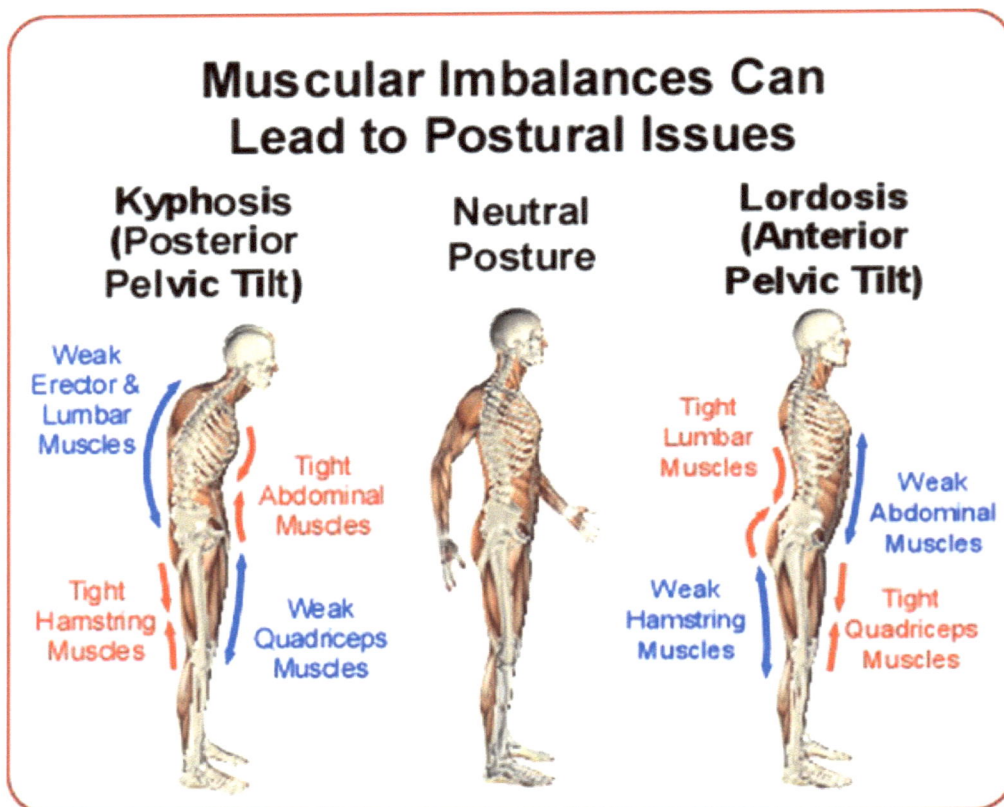

Muscular Imbalances Can Lead to Postural Issues

www.MindandBodyExercises.com

One Part Affects All Parts

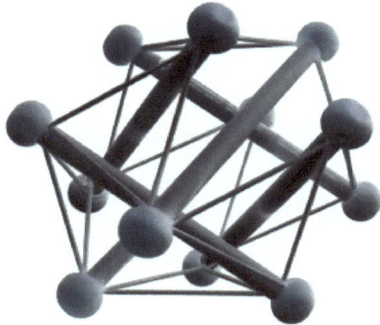

Just like the tensegrity model, tension on one area of the body can affect tension on all components throughout the human body.

Posture affects the nervous, muscular, circulatory & skeletal systems

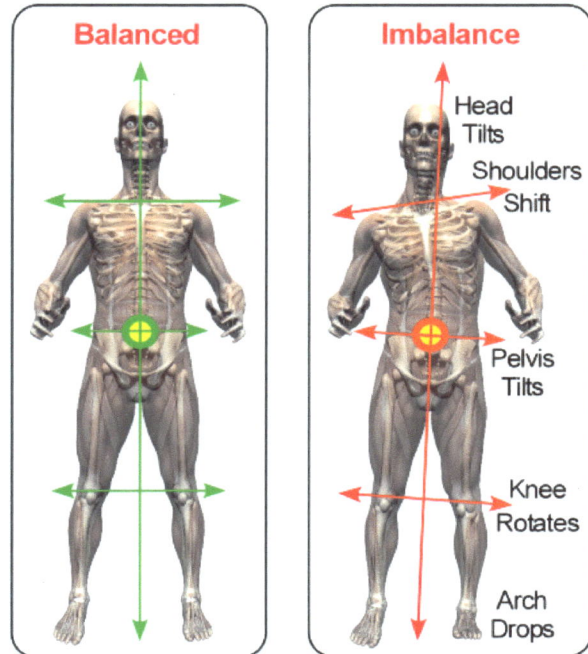

The Kinetic Chain

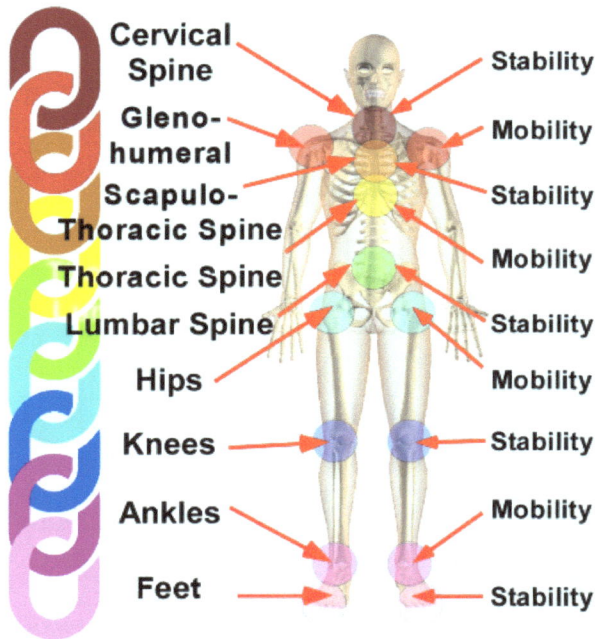

Cervical Spine	Stability
Gleno-humeral	Mobility
Scapulo-Thoracic Spine	Stability
Thoracic Spine	Mobility
Lumbar Spine	Stability
Hips	Mobility
Knees	Stability
Ankles	Mobility
Feet	Stability

Balanced

Imbalance
- Head Tilts
- Shoulders Shift
- Pelvis Tilts
- Knee Rotates
- Arch Drops

www.MindAndBodyExercises.com

"When one part is affected, all parts are affected"

Instinctively, as humans we try to center our head directly above our physical center of gravity. Poor posture, short leg syndrome, injuries or habitual body movements can cause remodeling of the muscular, skeletal and nervous system.

These root problems can be the cause of many chronic ailments. A difference in leg length by 7mm or 0.275″ can be enough to throw an individual's spine out of "calibration".

Shoulder pain can occur when one's side of the body is higher or lower than the opposite side.

Neck pain and headaches can occur when one side of the neck has more tension than the opposite.

Knee, hip and iliotibial band pain can occur when one's body weight is unevenly distributed between the two legs.

Knee pain can occur when one's body weight is unevenly distributed between the two legs.

Ankle pain can occur when one's side of the body is favored due to chronic pain

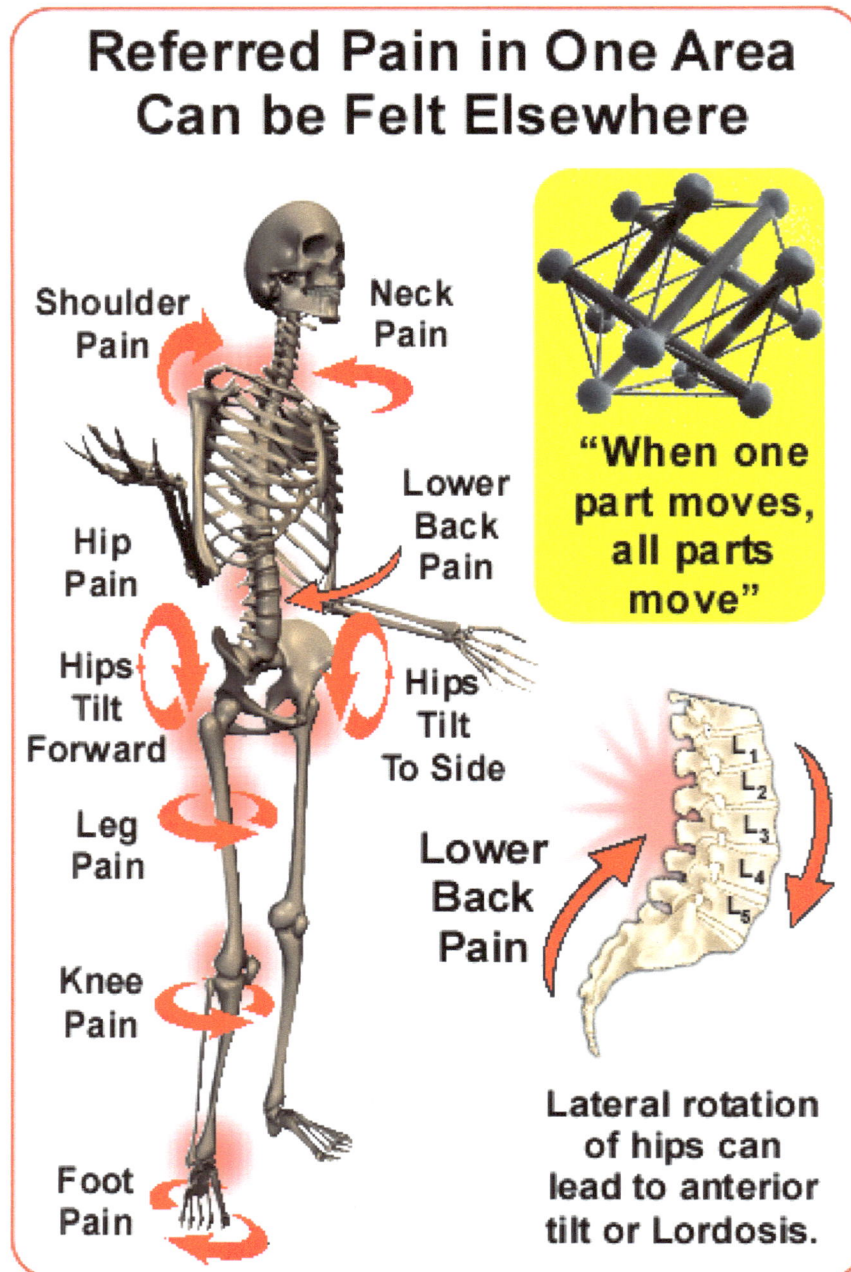

www.MindandBodyExercises.com

In 2019, 20.4% of adults had chronic pain and 7.4% of adults had chronic pain that frequently limited life or work activities (referred to as high impact chronic pain) in the past 3 months. Chronic pain and high-impact chronic pain both increased with age and were highest among adults aged 65 and over.

Non-Hispanic white adults (23.6%) were more likely to have chronic pain compared with non-Hispanic black (19.3%), Hispanic (13.0%), and non-Hispanic Asian (6.8%) adults.
Source: https://www.cdc.gov/nchs/products/databriefs/db390.htm

From my experience of over 40 years of martial arts, fitness and wellness training and teaching, I have seen some amazing benefits coming from qigong (yoga), tai chi any many other methods that are considered as "alternative". For those in fairly good shape, one can develop an amazing amount of strength throughout the whole body, but in particular the wrists, forearms, shoulders, lower back and legs. I have also trained individuals that have had more serious issues such as cerebral palsy, knee injuries, severe trauma to the spine and hip and other ailments that have shown great improvement.

Methods to Improve Imbalances

Course of Action:
- consult with your physician or chiropractor
- have your posture checked
- stretch regularly
- perform non-specific symmetrical exercises
- inspect footwear for uneven wear patterns
- evaluate poor posture habits and adjust
- review career choices if necessary

There are many individual exercises and techniques, that can stretch and release tension of the fascia trains throughout the human body. Tai Chi, Qigong, Yoga and Pilates are methods of stretching and strengthening the fascia as preventative or post-injury low impact exercises.

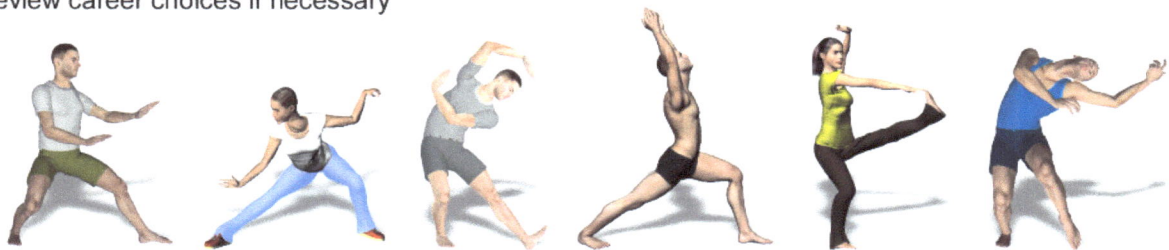

www.MindAndBodyExercises.com

© Copyright 2021 - CAD Graphics, Inc.

Kinetic linking is a widely known concept, not only relative to health and injuries but also for sports, athletics, martial arts and others. When a cowboy cracks a whip, kinetic linking is what makes the whip crack. Kinetic linking is what allows a baseball pitcher to deliver a 90-mph pitch, where kinetic linking allows the batter to hit the ball out of the park. In martial arts, it is this concept that lets a much smaller and seemingly weaker individual defend themselves effectively against a much stronger opponent. An example of this would be hitting someone in the nose with an open hand, while sitting at a table, versus the same person standing up and taking two steps forward while winding up their arm. Then stepping forward while extending their arm, like that whip to the aggressor's nose.

Kinetic Linking (the key to extraordinary power)

Kinetic - pertaining to movement or motion   **Linking** - to connect, unite

Cracking a bullwhip, exemplifies the physical action of kinetic linking. Not only does the whip accumulate speed and power, but the practitioner actually initiates the action beginning at the feet. A wave of movement throughout the bones and muscles, drives the momentum upwards and eventually is released through the wrist and hand.

Kinetic Linking is a common phenomenon occurring in baseball (batting & pitching), boxing, discus throwing as well as other sports and activities.

Many martial artists have known for hundreds of years, that kinetic linking is a key factor in developing power for self defense skills as well as a way of improving overall fitness.

The tip of the bullwhip can gain speeds at roughly 30 times the speed of the wave moving throughout the body, one can start to see the tremendous amount of speed and power that can be generated.

Types of Energy used in Kinetic Linking

Potential Energy - stored energy awaiting a use

Kinetic Energy - energy due to motion

Gravitational Force - objects attraction to one another

Centrifugal Energy - outward force on an object moving on a curve around another object
A spring can possess not only centrifugal energy, but also potential (waiting to unwind) and kinetic energy, as it unwinds.

Methods Used Within Traditional Chinese Medicine

One of the various methods often prescribed in TCM is exercise/movement. Meditation, Tai chi and qigong are methods that affect the breathing patterns which in Western medicine would be connected to stimulation of the vagus nerve and the parasympathetic nervous system. TCM recognizes these methods as a way to balance the qi in the energy meridians and consequently the organs. Management of the breath while practicing these methods is a way to balance emotion and psychological issues.

Various TCM methods of pain management:

- Acupuncture: very fine needles placed gently in the skin
- Acupressure, reflexology and/or massage
- Cupping: heated cups that create suction on your skin
- Herbs: teas, powders, and capsules made mostly from plants
- Meditation: a way to sit quietly and calm your mind
- Moxibustion: dried herbs burned near the skin
- Tai chi/qigong; exercises with slow movements and focus on the breath

Some Options to Manage Pain
www.MindAndBodyExercises.com

Western Methods

Pain Relievers
Non-opiod pain medicines such as Acetaminophen, Ibuprofen, Naproxen

Antidepressants and Anticonvulsants
Medications that also have benefits for treating depression and seizures

Exercise
Exercise and physical therapy have been known to ease pain symptoms

Cognitive Behavioral Therapy
Managing thoughts and behaviors related to pain

Ancient Eastern Exercise Methods

Tai Chi
Slow moving yoga-type exercises with rhythmic breathing and self-awareness of mind & body.

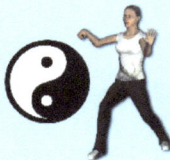

BaguaZhang
Walking Meditation or "walking of the circle" are all names for this style of Kung Fu training. An internal developing style similar to Tai Chi. Bagua develops stability in motion amongst many other things.

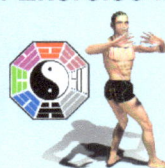

Qigong
Breathing exercises, with little or no body movement. When the mind is relaxed, the body chemistry changes and promotes natural healing.

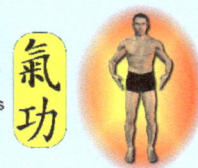

氣功

Other Methods Using Reflexology, Energy Meridians and/or Specific Strategic Trauma

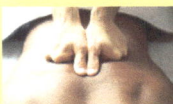

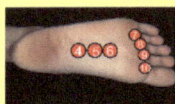

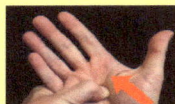

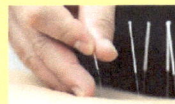

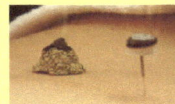

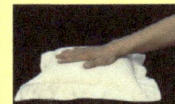

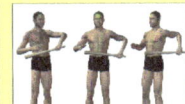

Massage	Reflexology	Acupressure	Acupuncture	Moxibustion	Iron Palm	Iron Body
General or specific manipulation by pressure upon the various muscles throughout the human body.	Application of specific pressure to the feet, hands or ears to stimulate energy throughout the body.	Manipulation of various "pressure points" throughout the body that connect to the energy meridians.	Similar to acupressure but using very thin needles to stimulate energy flow within the energy meridians.	Burning of dried mugwort on specific acupuncture points with or without the use of fine needles.	Precise conditioning techniques typically meant to condition the hands by hitting specific acupressure or reflexology points upon the hands.	Similar to Iron Palm conditioning techniques typically but hitting specific acupressure or reflexology points throughout the whole body.

These methods are all part of the same branch of knowledge of our internal energy flow to enhance longevity or relieve blockages within the human body.

The Role of Tai Chi, Qigong, and Breath Management

Stroke is a major cause of long-term disability, affecting millions globally. Conventional rehabilitation methods focus primarily on physical and cognitive therapy. However, mind-body practices like Tai Chi, Qigong, and breath regulation have emerged as effective complementary interventions. This article explores the physiological and psychological benefits of these practices in post-stroke recovery, supported by peer-reviewed evidence and recent clinical studies.

A stroke occurs when blood flow to the brain is interrupted, leading to a range of impairments in movement, speech, memory, and emotional regulation. Recovery can be slow and incomplete, with many survivors experiencing long-term disability. While conventional stroke rehabilitation includes physical therapy, speech-language therapy, and occupational therapy, integrating holistic practices like Tai Chi, Qigong, and breathwork has been researched and may significantly enhance outcomes (Li et al., 2012; Wang et al., 2022).

INTEGRATIVE MIND–BODY PRACTICES IN STROKE REHABILITATION

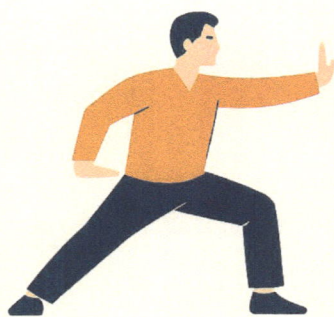

TAI CHI
- Improves balance & mobility
- Enhances daily functioning
- Supports neuroplasticity

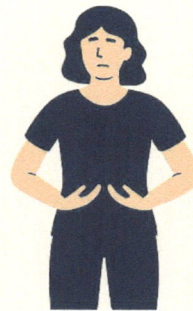

QIGONG
- Reduces muscle spasticity
- Boosts quality of life
- Fosters resilience

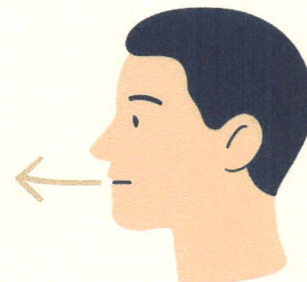

BREATH MANAGEMENT
- Aids neurological recovery
- Decreases stress
- Optimizes pulmonary function

Tai Chi for Stroke Recovery

Tai Chi is a low-impact, meditative exercise rooted in Chinese martial arts, consisting of slow, flowing movements coordinated with breath and focused attention. Studies indicate Tai Chi is safe and beneficial for stroke survivors, particularly for improving balance, mobility, and activities of daily living (ADLs) (Park et al., 2022).

In a meta-analysis of 27 randomized controlled trials involving 1,919 stroke survivors, Tai Chi was found to significantly improve dynamic balance (Hedges' g = 1.04), walking ability (Hedges' g = 0.81), and ADL performance (Hedges' g = 0.43) (Park et al., 2022). Additionally, seated Tai Chi adaptations demonstrated improved upper-limb function and mental health, making it ideal for those with limited mobility (American Heart Association [AHA], 2022).

Furthermore, Tai Chi supports postural control by engaging both the musculoskeletal and nervous systems, promoting neuroplasticity, an essential component in recovery after stroke-induced brain damage (Li et al., 2012).

Qigong as a Therapeutic Modality

Qigong integrates movement, breathing, and mental focus to cultivate "qi" or vital life energy. Like Tai Chi, it is accessible, adaptable, and especially effective in promoting both physical and psychological healing in stroke patients (Wang et al., 2022).

Qigong has been shown to reduce muscle spasticity, improve upper and lower limb function, and enhance the quality of life in stroke survivors. Moreover, it fosters mental resilience, helping to reduce depression and anxiety, two common post-stroke complications (Wang et al., 2022).

To substantiate the claim about the adaptability of Qigong for individuals at all recovery stages, you can refer to the study by Wang et al. (2022), which highlights Qigong's effectiveness in promoting physical and psychological healing for stroke patients. This research emphasizes Qigong's versatility, as it can be practiced in various postures of standing, seated, or lying down, making it suitable for diverse mobility levels.

Breath Management Techniques

Breath control plays a foundational role in both Tai Chi and Qigong, but it also serves as a stand-alone therapy in stroke rehabilitation. Breathing exercises like diaphragmatic breathing, pursed-lip breathing, and alternate nostril breathing improve pulmonary function, reduce stress, and enhance neurological recovery (Kang et al., 2022)

A recent review by Kang (2022) found that stroke patients engaging in structured breathwork showed measurable improvements in cognitive function and mental alertness. Controlled breathing can modulate the autonomic nervous system, reduce sympathetic arousal, and improve oxygen delivery to brain tissue. These are crucial factors for healing post-stroke. Another meta-analysis found that respiratory muscle training significantly improved walking ability, respiratory strength, and vital capacity in stroke survivors (Liu et al., 2024). Breath regulation also fosters mindfulness and can reduce stress-induced cortisol levels, which otherwise impair cognitive and physical recovery.

BREATHWORK FOR STROKE REHABILITATION

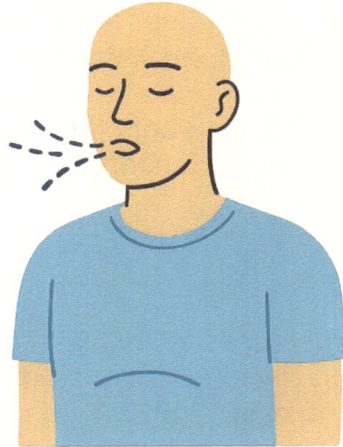

DIAPHRAGMATIC BREATHING

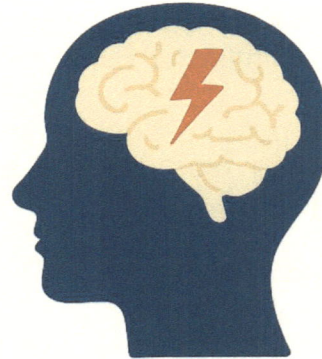

- Improves cognitive function
- Modulates nervous system
- Reduces stress

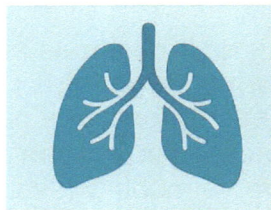

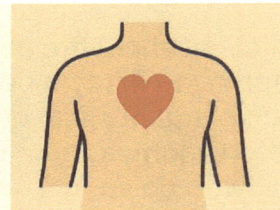

PULMONARY FUNCTION   **MINDFULNESS**   **PHYSICAL RECOVERY**

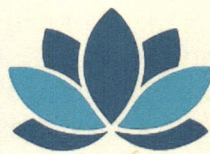

Clinical Integration and Application

The integration of Tai Chi, Qigong, and breath management into stroke rehabilitation offers a complementary model that addresses the whole person: body, mind, and spirit. These practices are particularly suited for long-term maintenance and chronic stroke management because they are low-cost, non-invasive, and patient empowering.

Rehabilitation professionals can incorporate these practices as part of a tiered recovery program. For instance, seated Qigong or Tai Chi can be introduced early, with progression toward standing forms as the patient's balance and strength improve. Breath training may be applied across all stages, helping regulate mood and improve mental clarity from the onset (Wang et al., 2022).

Instructor certification and training should be considered when implementing these practices in clinical settings to ensure safety and efficacy. Additionally, ongoing research is warranted to explore the neurological mechanisms by which these practices influence post-stroke plasticity and rehabilitation outcomes.

Conclusion

Tai Chi, Qigong, and breath management represent powerful, evidence-based adjuncts to conventional stroke rehabilitation. These mind-body practices enhance physical recovery, cognitive function, emotional well-being, and spiritual resilience. By fostering neuroplasticity, emotional regulation, and functional independence, they provide a holistic and empowering pathway for stroke survivors. Integrating these modalities into clinical care can support a more complete and compassionate recovery journey.

References:

American Heart Association. (2022, April 7). *Seated form of tai chi might boost stroke recovery.* https://www.heart.org/en/news/2022/04/07/seated-form-of-tai-chi-might-boost-stroke-recovery

Li, F., Harmer, P., Fitzgerald, K., Eckstrom, E., Stock, R., Galver, J., Maddalozzo, G., & Batya, S. S. (2012). Tai Chi and postural stability in patients with Parkinson's disease. *New England Journal of Medicine, 366*(6), 511–519. https://doi.org/10.1056/NEJMoa1107911

Liu, Y., Liu, X., Liu, Y., Zhang, L., Zhang, L., Wang, J., Shi, Y., & Xie, Q. (2024). Effects of respiratory muscle training on post-stroke rehabilitation: A systematic review and meta-analysis. *World Journal of Clinical Cases*, *12*(20), 4289–4300. https://doi.org/10.12998/wjcc.v12.i20.4289

Park, M., Song, R., Ju, K., Seo, J., Fan, X., Ryu, A., Li, L., & Kim, J. (2022). Effects of Tai Chi and Qigong on the mobility of stroke survivors: A systematic review and meta-analysis of randomized trials. *PLOS ONE, 17*(11), e0277541. https://doi.org/10.1371/journal.pone.0277541

Wang, Y., Zhang, Q., Li, F., Li, Q., & Jin, Y. (2022). Effects of tai chi and Qigong on cognition in neurological disorders: A systematic review and meta-analysis. *Geriatric Nursing, 46*, 166–177. https://doi.org/10.1016/j.gerinurse.2022.05.014

Yang, H., Li, B., Feng, L., Zhang, Z., & Liu, X. (2023). Effects of health Qigong exercise on upper extremity muscle activity, balance function, and quality of life in stroke patients. *Frontiers in Neuroscience, 17*, 1208554. https://doi.org/10.3389/fnins.2023.1208554

Kang, E. S., Yook, J. S., & Ha, M. S. (2022). Breathing Exercises for Improving Cognitive Function in Patients with Stroke. *Journal of clinical medicine*, *11*(10), 2888. https://doi.org/10.3390/jcm11102888

A key concept in relieving pain is to increase flexibility (range of motion) while building strength, to provide stability and support in the injured areas.

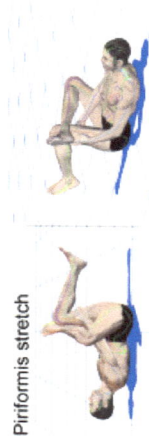

A key concept in relieving pain is to increase flexibility (range of motion) while building strength, to provide stability and support in the injured areas.

Torso twist
Sit on the buttocks with one leg straight and one leg bent and crossed over the other. Turn the upper body opposite while relaxing the back.

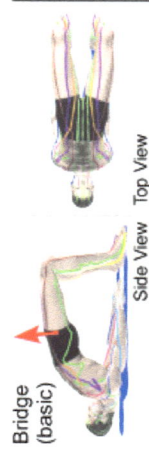

Bridge (basic)
Side View   Top View
Lay flat on the back, push hips upward as keeping shoulders and feet on the ground.

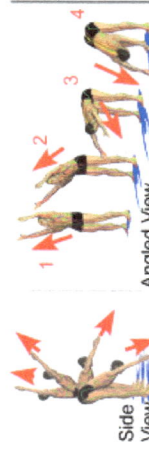

Side View   Angled View
Can be held for intervals of time at different angles of height or continuously stretching as bending forward.

Cat Tilt
Top View   Side View
Rest on hands and knees as pulling stomach and lower back upwards while pulling chin in towards the chest.

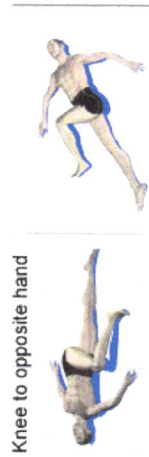

Knee to opposite hand
Lay flat on your back, bring a bent knee across the other straight leg. Relax the neck and arms as you feel the lower back stretch to the side.

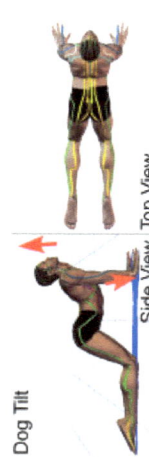

Dog Tilt
Top View   Side View
Rest on hands and knees as pulling stomach and lower back downwards while pulling chin upwards.

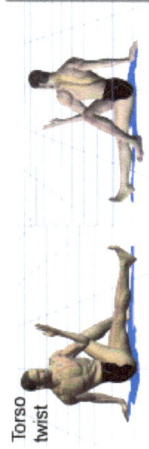

Piriformis stretch
Lay flat on the back as bending both knees. Try to cross the right foot over the left knee. Pull the left leg towards your face as the right hip stretches.

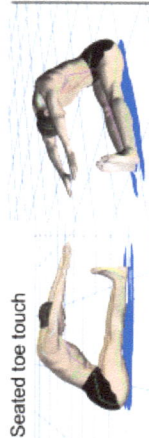

Seated toe touch
Sit on the buttocks as leaning the upper body forward. Focus more on the torso coming forward than the hands reaching the feet.

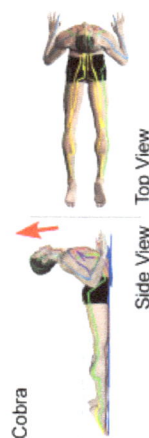

Cobra
Top View   Side View
Lay flat on the stomach while pushing the hands downward and the head and shoulders upward.

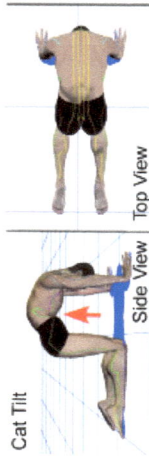

Try to match your body position similar to those as shown. Don't be discouraged by not being able to achieve these stretches but rather do what your body is capable of. Stretches can be performed on the floor, on a mattress or even in a swimming pool or hot tub. Try for a few seconds in each position for a total of a few minutes. As your flexibility increases in the hamstrings, less tension will be placed on the lower back muscles. Use discretion when attempting any exercise that may cause pain or further discomfort. Exercises where the back is arched forward should be practiced with extreme caution and patience.

Attempt to do some of the exercises every day for at least a few days in a row. As the pain is relieved, try to add more time for each exercise working up to a total of a half-hour or full hour. As less pain is present, try to maintain a regular schedule of performing these exercises to keep the problem from recurring. All stretches should be performed on both sides. Relax the body into the positions in spite of any tension in the muscles. Deep and relaxed breathing (qigong) is essential while performing these exercises.

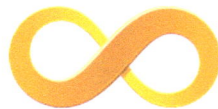

Back Pain Management

Most people in the United States will experience back pain at some time in their lives. Causes of back pain are many, ranging from poor posture, heavy lifting, and lack of exercise among other issues. Some may find relief through chiropractic or acupuncture therapy. Depending upon the root cause, most pain goes away within a few days or weeks, only to return at a later date. Unless the root cause is fixed, most treatments only offer temporary relief. In many cases, the root cause of back pain is tight hamstring muscles and/or poor posture. Excessive sitting can tighten these muscles as well as a lack of proper stretching on a regular basis contribute to many back pain issues. How we sit, how we stand and how we move, or more often don't move – all affect our posture and relative issues with the spine and the nervous system.

Not having back pain, does not necessarily mean your spine is in great shape! If not disease or illness is a goal, we need to focus on being fit, well & healthy. Good health usually comes at a cost of time, effort, sacrifice and resources, or a combination of the prior. Most people don't care to make the investment into taking care of themselves until after they are injured. Even then, most people with back issues often choose pain medicines or sometimes surgery over exercise or lifestyle changes that can improve their situation. Traumatic injuries are often best treated with emergency surgery and that is really not the topic of this post.

In 2019, 20.4% of adults had chronic pain and 7.4% of adults had chronic pain that frequently limited life or work activities (referred to as high impact chronic pain) in the past 3 months. Chronic pain and high-impact chronic pain both increased with age and were highest among adults aged 65 and over.

Non-Hispanic white adults (23.6%) were more likely to have chronic pain compared with non-Hispanic black (19.3%), Hispanic (13.0%), and non-Hispanic Asian (6.8%) adults.
Source: https://www.cdc.gov/nchs/products/databriefs/db390.htm

Addressing the root problems of back pain can affect our health and well-being. There are many methods available to manage back pain without pharmaceuticals, nor surgery when at all possible. Yoga, qigong, tai chi, martial arts, Traditional Chinese Medicine, reflexology/acupressure, deep breathing, meditation and other methods are all possible options upon individual circumstances.

What may be helpful are many exercises and methods that develop strength and flexibility, which improve posture and relative spine health. Good health of the entire spinal structure starts with good posture. Strength in the back, hips and abdomen provide a strong cage that houses the internal organs. Flexibility in these areas helps to maintain good blood circulation to the organs and lower body. Lengthening of the spine while exercising reduces stress and tension on the nervous system. Additionally, exercises that promote deep and relaxed breathing can help manage stress and pain. These can be practiced while performing the back exercises or as stand-alone methods.

Relieve Sciatica & Lower Back Pain

Sciatica can be more painful and debilitating than the occasional strain or pulled muscle. Causes of back pain can be many ranging from poor posture, heavy lifting, sports injuries and lack of exercise among others. Most muscle pain goes away within a few days or weeks but sciatica can be an ongoing chronic symptom of a more serious condition requiring extra attention. Unless the root cause is fixed, most treatments only offer temporary relief. In many cases, the root cause of back pain is tight hamstring muscles. Excessive sitting can tighten these muscles as well as lack of activity on a regular basis. The set of exercises on page 2 of this graphic, lengthen, strengthen and increase flexibility within the spine, which improve posture. These are key factors with sciatica as the vertebrae can pinch the nerve roots.

Symptoms of Sciatica:
- pain in lower back, hips, legs and/or feet
- burning, tingling, numbness, weakness

Causes of Sciatica:
- disc herniation
- bone spurs
- postural imbalances
- tight muscular structure
- obesity
- injury

Treatments:
- rest
- chiropractic
- exercise
- surgery
- pain meds
- massage
- therapy
- acupuncture

Dermatomes Show the Connection of the Spine, Nerves and Skin Throughout the Body

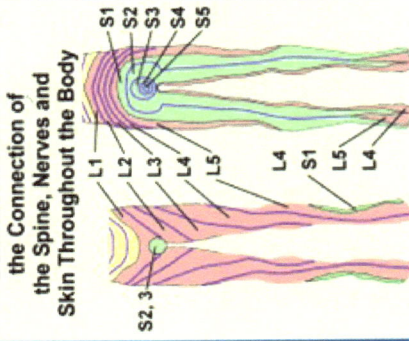

Lumbar Nerve Roots
Sciatic Nerve

L4
L5
Sacrum
Disc Herniation

Sacral Plexus and the Sciatic Nerve
L4
L5
S1
S2
S3
(posterior view)

Just like the tensegrity model, tension on one area, can affect tension on all components throughout the structure.

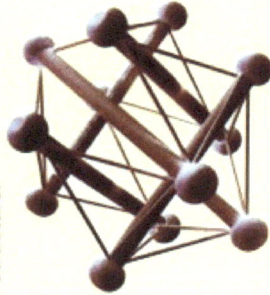

Posture & Symmetry

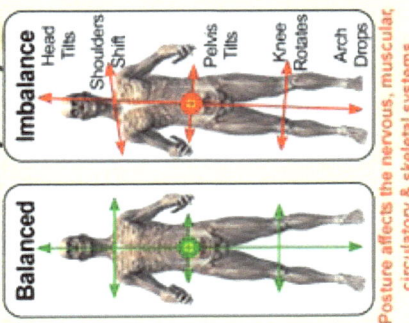

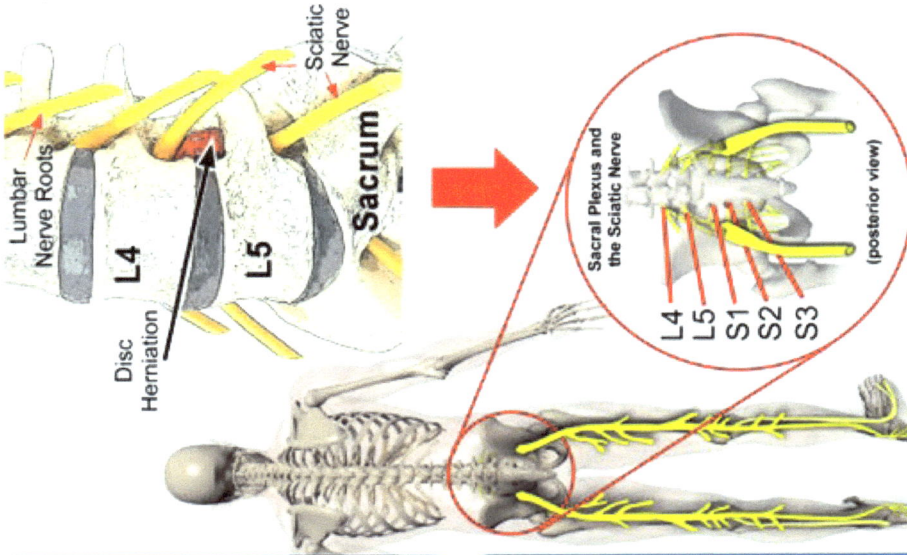

Balanced

Imbalance
Head Tilts
Shoulders Shift
Pelvis Tilts
Knee Rotates
Arch Drops

Posture affects the nervous, muscular, circulatory & skeletal systems

Compressed Spine Can Affect Other Areas

The health of the spine affects the nervous, muscular, circulatory & skeletal systems

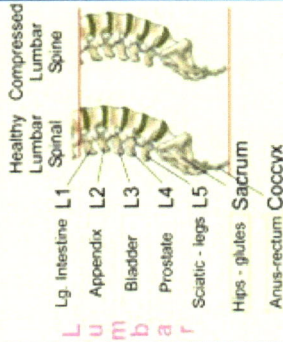

Healthy Lumbar Spinal
Compressed Lumbar Spine

L1 - Lg. Intestine
L2 - Appendix
L3 - Bladder
L4 - Prostate
L5 - Sciatic - legs
Sacrum - Hips - glutes
Coccyx - Anus-rectum

Nerve Root Issues

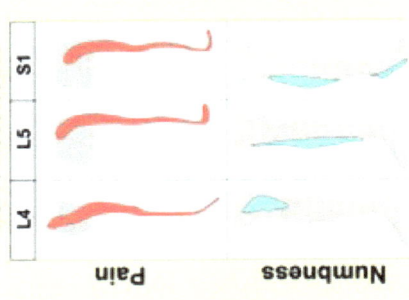

L4	L5	S1

Pain
Numbness

S1
S2
S3
S4
S5
L1
L2
L3
L4
L5
L4
S1
L5
L4
S2, 3

How to Build Strong Bones

Often people seek Western medicine (also known as allopathic or biomedicine) and its strong usage of pharmaceuticals to manage bone density and relative ailments of osteopenia and osteoporosis. I have discussed in other posts about the link to how the autonomic nervous system manages stress, blood chemistry and relative physiological organ functions. However, this post will address more on how the root cause of all types of disease and illness, being the lack of physical weight-bearing activities.

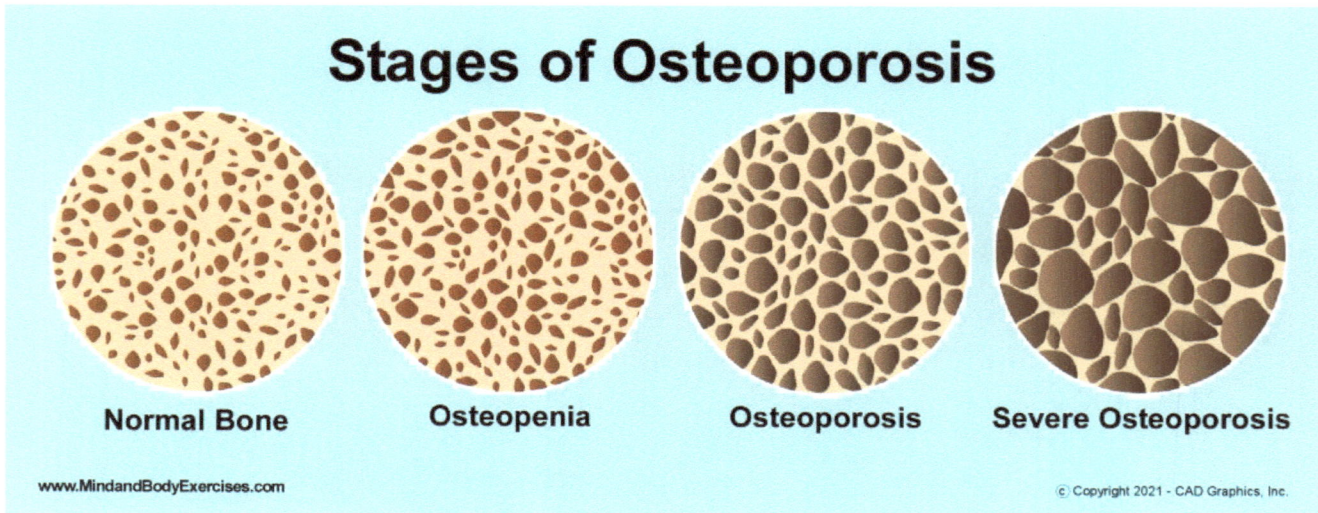

Stages of Osteoporosis — Normal Bone, Osteopenia, Osteoporosis, Severe Osteoporosis

www.MindandBodyExercises.com © Copyright 2021 - CAD Graphics, Inc.

The joints of our body are composed of two or more bones joining together, along with the muscles, tendons, cartilage, synovium and ligaments that hold the whole structure together. The shape of our bones reflects the forces applied to them. For example, small bumps, ridges and other features on the surface of our bones are the attachment sites for tendons.

When muscles are put under more load through activities, stress or exercises, the corresponding attachment sites enlarge to withstand the increased forces. Bones that are under more stress become thicker and stronger, while in contrast bones that are not subjected to ordinary stresses tend to become weaker, thin and more brittle. Wolff's law, developed by anatomist & surgeon Julius Wolff in the 19th century, states that "bone in a healthy person or animal will adapt to the loads under which it is placed."

By engaging our bones with strategic trauma exercise methods (or specific stress without injury) that can be regulated by the individual to make bones stronger and prevent osteopenia and/or osteoporosis. These types of exercises fall into 3 different categories of tension, impact and vibration exercises. Ironically, while some of these methods improve bone and muscular strength, they sometimes can cause pain and injury to the same joints that the individual might be trying to strengthen. Fox example, jumping rope, hiking and tennis might cause more injury to a 60+ than the benefits that might be gained from these practices.

Wolff's Law

Wolff's Law states that our bones become thicker and stronger over time to resist forces placed upon them and thinner and weaker if there are no forces to act against. Wolff's Law and Injury. This principle is important for preventing injuries. A thicker bone is harder to break.

Tension and compression cycles create a small electrical potential that stimulates bone deposition and increased density at points of stress.

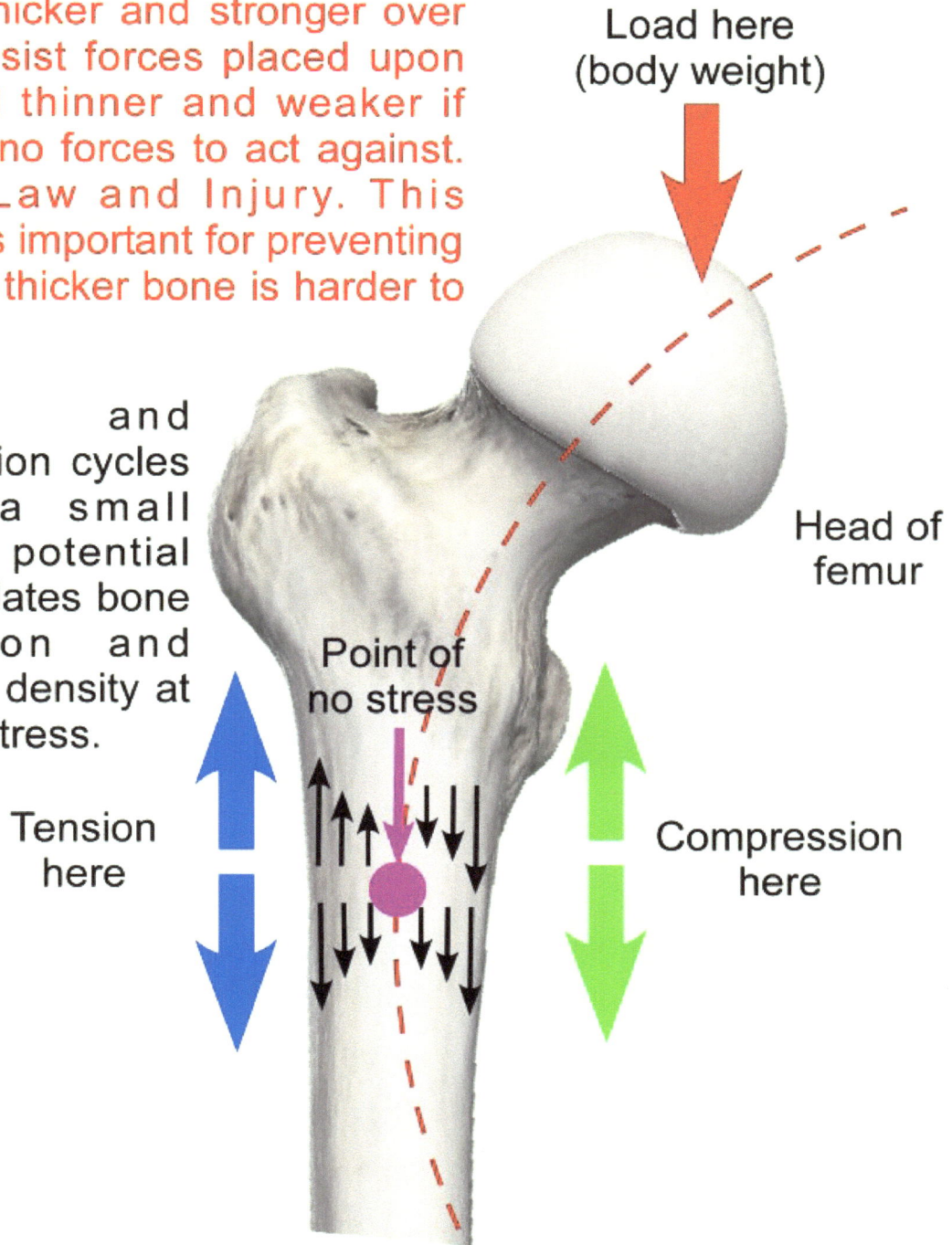

Load here
(body weight)

Head of femur

Point of no stress

Tension here

Compression here

Regular weight-bearing exercise is an important component for maintaining healthy bone structure. Avid weightlifters often have thick bones with very prominent ridges. Non-athletes or those who have little to moderate physical activity will find weight-bearing activities are imperative for stimulating normal bone metabolism of maintenance as well as maintaining bone strength. Below are some examples of weight-bearing exercises that require very little equipment beyond one's own body weight. Proper instruction is recommended over learning from a graphic, book or video.

EXERCISE METHODS USING STRATEGIC TRAUMA:

TENSION	IMPACT	VIBRATION
Dancing	Aerobics	Machine therapy
Elastic Bands	Hiking	Tapping methods
Qigong (Chi Kung)	Jump rope	
Pilates	Running	
Stair-Step machine	Stair climbing	
Tai Chi	Tennis	
Treadmill	Walking - brisk	
Weights		
Yard Work		
Yoga	www.MindAndBodyExercises.com	

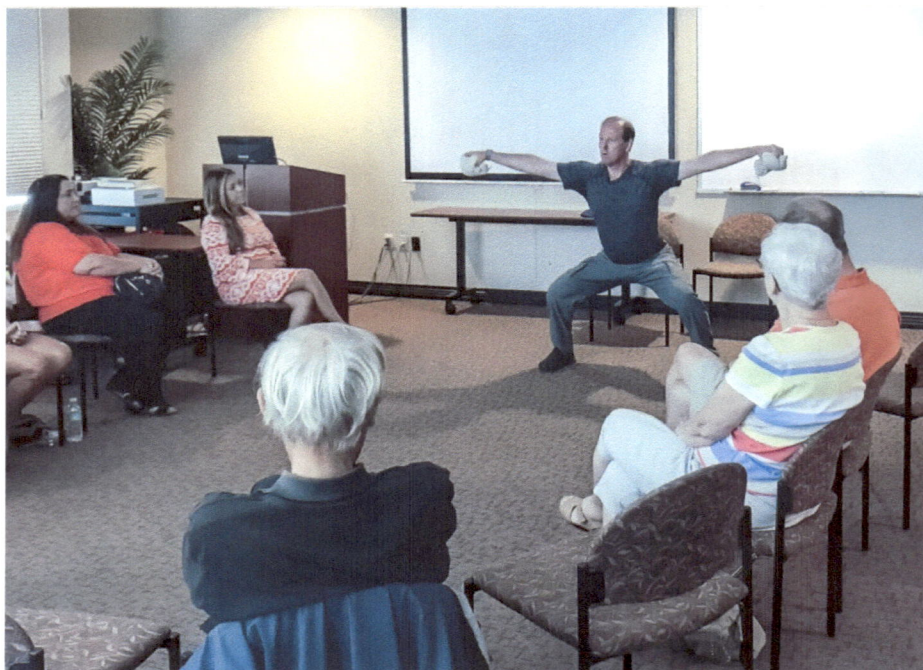

Shim Yuk - Whole Body Engagement

The nervous system innervates the muscles that are engaged during practice of the Shim Yuk exercises. Additionally, the cardiopulmonary and skeletal systems are also engaged. Focused thought is necessary in order to maintain the correct posture while executing each repetition.

Cervical Muscles:
sternocleidomastoid
scalenus
spinalis cervicis
spinalis capitus
semispinalis cervicis
semispinalis capitus
splenius cervicis
longus colli cervicis
longus capitus

rectus capitus anterior
rectus capitus lateralis
Iliocostalis cervicis
longissimus cervicis
longissimus capitis
rectus capitus posterior major
rectus capitus posterior minor
obliquus capitus Inferior
obliquus capitus superior

Shoulder, Arm & Chest Muscles:
infraspinatus
triceps brachii
pectoralis major
pectoralis minor
teres major
biceps brachii
latissimus dorsi
subscapularis
supraspinatus

Hand & Wrist Muscles:
abductor digiti minimi
abductor pollicis brevis
abductor pollicis longus
adductor pollicis
brachioradialis
dorsal expansion (hood)
dorsal Interosseous
extensor carpi radialis brevis
extensor carpi radialis longus
extensor carpi ulnaris
extensor digiti minimi
extensor digitorum
extensor Indicis
extensor pollicis brevis
extensor retinaculum
flexor carpi radialis
flexor carpi ulnaris
flexor digiti minimi brevis
flexor digitorum profundus
flexor digitorum superficialis
flexor pollicis brevis
flexor retinaculum
lumbrical muscles
opponens pollicis
palmar Interosseous
palmaris longus
pronator quadratus

Thoracic Muscles:
longissimus thoracis
Iliocostalis thoracis
spinalis thoracis
semispinalis thoracis
rotatores thoracis

Muscles of the Buttocks:
gluteus maximus
gluteus medius
gluteus minimus

Quadricep Muscles:
rectus femoris,
vastus lateralis
vastus intermedius
vastus medialis

Lumbar Muscles:
psoas major
Intertransversarii lateralis
quadratus lumborum
Interspinales
Intertransversarii mediales
multifidus
longissimus lumborum
Iliocostalis lumborum

Hamstring Muscle Group:
semitendinosus
semimembranosus
biceps femoris

ankle muscles:
gastrocnemius
soleus
tibialis posterior
tibialis anterior
peroneus longus
peroneus brevis
flexor hallucis longus
flexor digitorum longus
extensor hallucis longus
extensor digitorum longus

Muscles of the Foot:
flexor hallucis brevis
abductor hallucis
flexor digitorum longus
lumbricals
flexor digitorum brevis
quadratus plantae

www.MindAndBodyExercises.com

Exercise #1

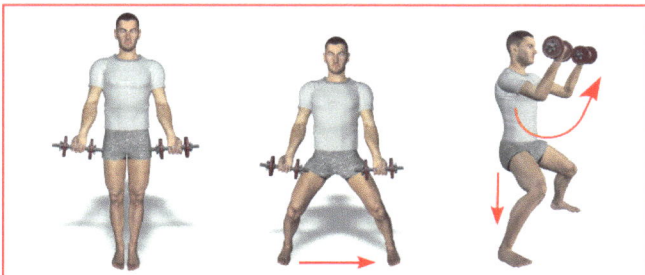

Start with dumbbells at thighs, palms forward. Step feet to double shoulder width apart. Drop the hips while keeping foot, knee and thigh within the same vertical plane. Raise hands up to eye-level by bending slowly from the elbows.

Exercise #2

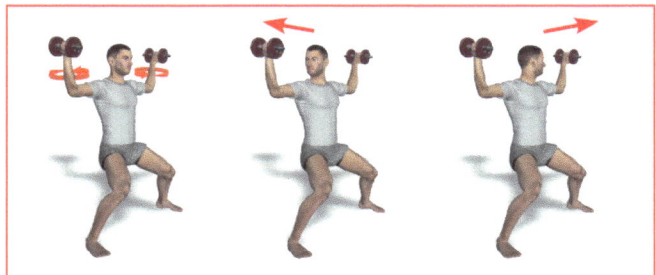

From previous position, rotate both wrists outward as turning head as far as possible to the right and then to the left. Again, drop the hips while keeping foot, knee and thigh within the same vertical plane. Exhale deeply as sinking the hips.

www.MindandBodyExercises.com

105

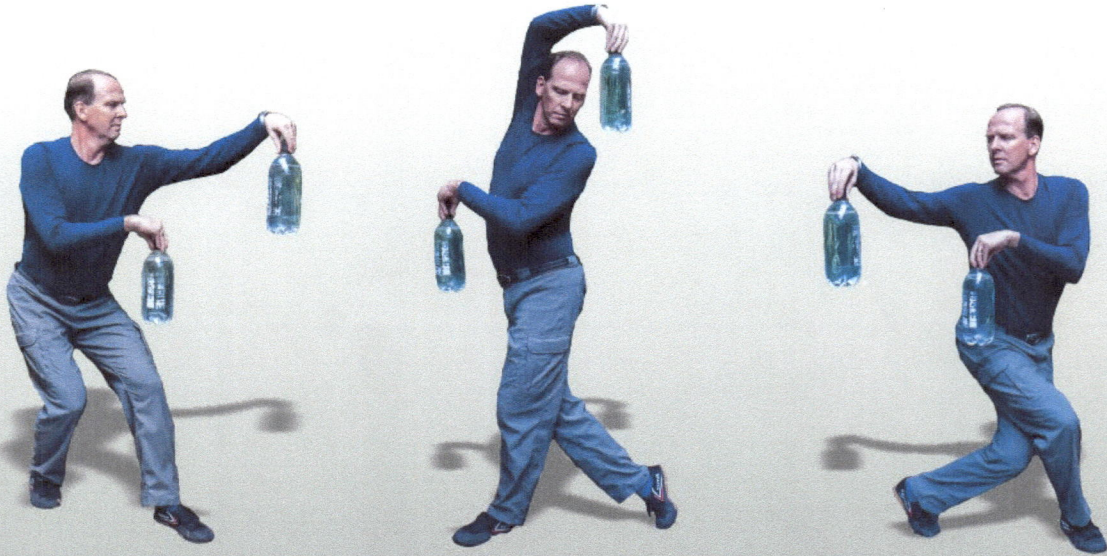

9 Major Joints · Muscular System · Circulatory System · Fascia Trains · Lymphatic System · Skeletal System · Nervous System

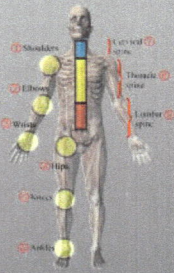

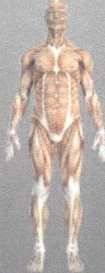

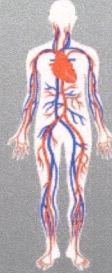

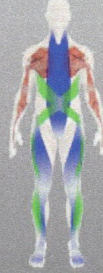

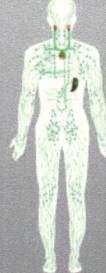

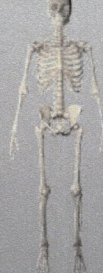

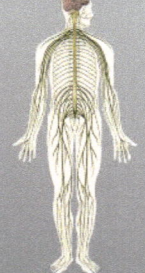

www.MindandBodyExercises.com

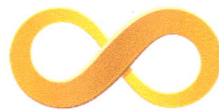

Fat in Our Diet – Friend or Foe?

Nutritional information has been evolving and accessible for decades, but we need to look to many diverse sources to find the most accurate information for any particular topic. Particular fats such as saturated, mono-saturated and polyunsaturated fats, all have specific health benefits when consumed in moderation. Saturated fats contain cholesterol that the cells within our bodies rely upon for structure and barriers.1 Over the last few decades, trans fats have been known to mostly have little or no positive health benefits.

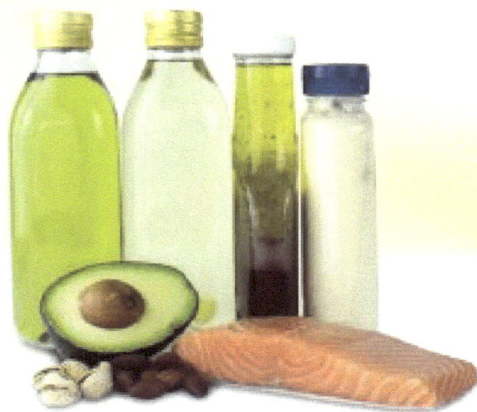 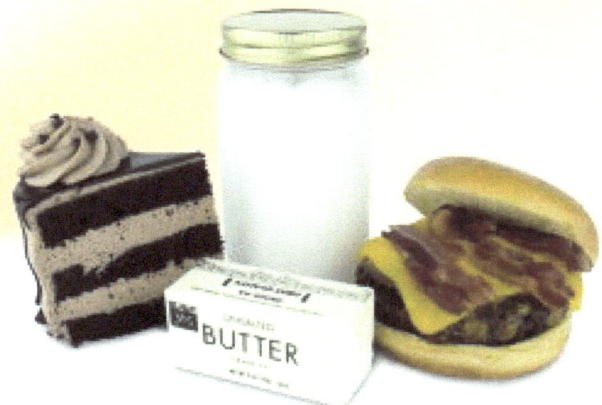

I think it so very important that we seek education in our personal nutrition as to become more aware of exactly what we are putting into our bodies. Over the last decades, consumers have relied upon the scientific and medical industries to inform the general public about what is healthy or unhealthy to consume. Depending on the source of the information, fat and consequently cholesterol are possibly the source of all of our health-related issues or the cure to all that ails us.1 Perhaps the truth lies somewhere in between and realizing that we as humans do need specific fats in our diet, albeit in moderation. Additionally, what may be deemed healthy or beneficial for someone, may not be for another. Everyone has their own health constitution relative to genetics, lifestyle, environment, and maybe other components.

We have seen phases or trends in US health culture evolve over time. We can rationalize this by realizing that science has continuously been evolving, and data has become more accurate due to many technological advances since the early part of the 20th century.

Unfortunately, many of the trends have been affected by big corporations and associations that have vast resources to sway not only the medical and science communities but also the public as well. Cigarettes were promoted by doctors, then they were not but the FDA still regulates and allows their detrimental usage.2 Coffee and its ingredient of caffeine seems to ebb and flow every year between being good or bad for us. 3 A few decades ago, eggs and beef were demonized as having little positive health benefits to outweigh their negative effects such as high cholesterol and relative higher risk of heart disease from high consumption.

1984

2014

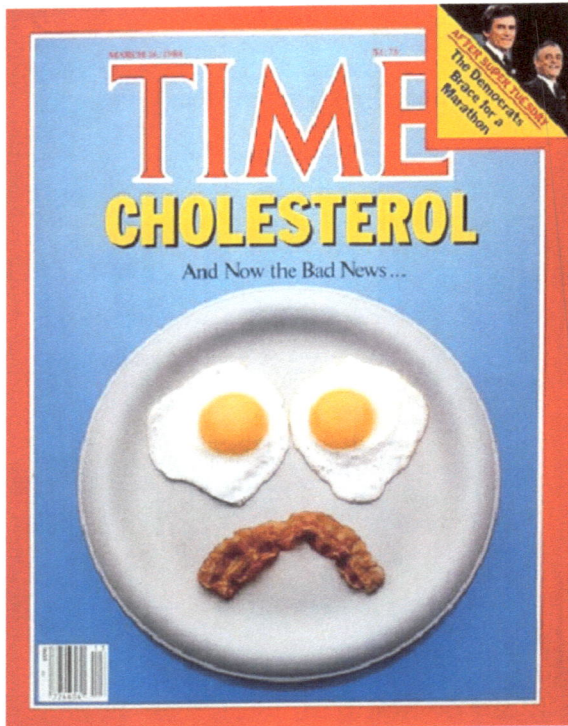

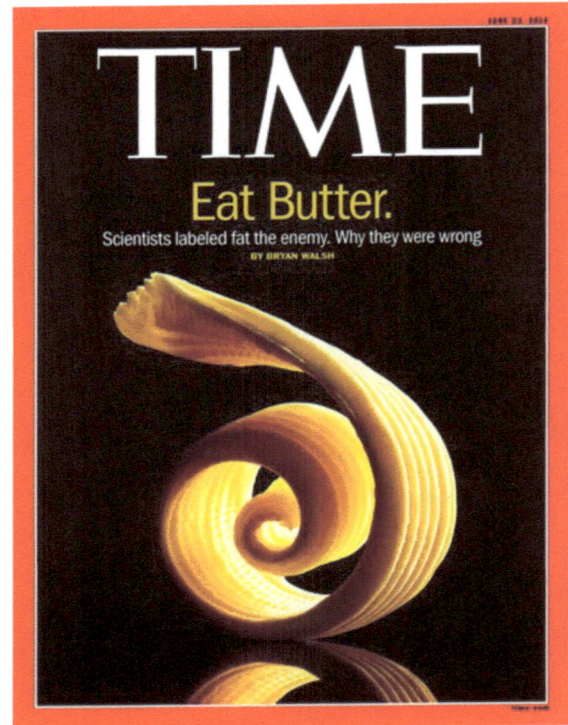

In the 70's a diet filled with eggs, bacon, beef, salt and sugar was desired as it was a symbol of social status to be able to afford these items and provide for one's family. I think this was a side effect of my parents' having grown up during the Great Depression, where jobs and food were somewhat limited. When I was a teen back in the 80's, I saw the beginning of the shift from the eggs, bacon and pancake breakfast and steak and potatoes dinners to an awareness that these foods were high in fat and relative cholesterol.

With my own pursuit of better health and well-being, I have found that nutrition is highly relative to the individual's lifestyle choices and awareness that even seemingly healthy foods may not be so much, especially if they have been heavily processed, contain pesticides or other chemicals added to them. So, I read labels more and consume in moderation.

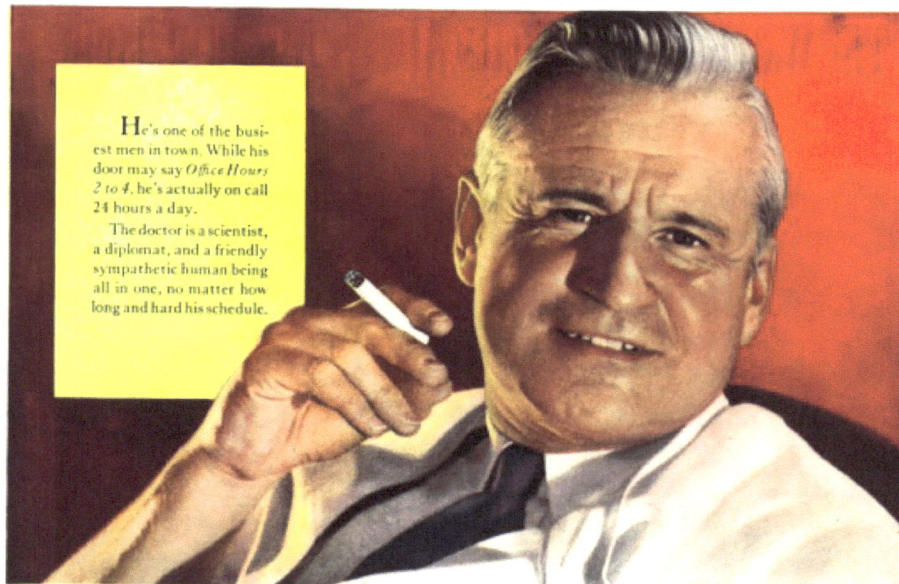

According to a recent Nationwide survey:

MORE DOCTORS SMOKE CAMELS THAN ANY OTHER CIGARETTE

DOCTORS in every branch of medicine — 113,597 in all — were queried in this nationwide study of cigarette preference. Three leading research organizations made the survey. The gist of the query was — What cigarette do you smoke, Doctor?

The brand named most was Camel!

The rich, full flavor and cool mildness of Camel's superb blend of costlier tobaccos seem to have the same appeal to the smoking tastes of doctors as to millions of other smokers. If you are a Camel smoker, this preference among doctors will hardly surprise you. If you're not — well, try Camels now.

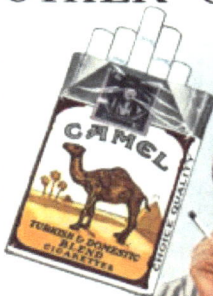

Your "T-Zone" Will Tell You...

T for Taste ...
T for Throat ...

that's your proving ground for any cigarette. See if Camels don't suit your "T-Zone" to a "T."

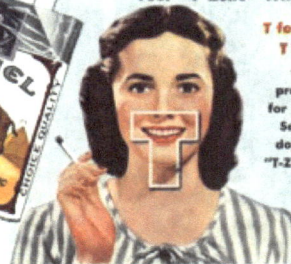

CAMELS *Costlier Tobaccos*

References:

[1] Campbell-McBride, N. (2017, November 6). Cholesterol: Friend Or Foe? The Weston A. Price Foundation. https://www.westonaprice.org/health-topics/know-your-fats/cholesterol-friend-or-foe/

[2] Little, B. (2020, January 8). When Cigarette Companies Used Doctors to Push Smoking. HISTORY. https://www.history.com/news/cigarette-ads-doctors-smoking-endorsement

[3] Is coffee good or bad for your health? (2021, April 9). News. https://www.hsph.harvard.edu/news/hsph-in-the-news/is-coffee-good-or-bad-for-your-health/

Many months have gone by with the world and the United States dealing with the COVID-19 pandemic. Much has been learned as more data has been compiled to determine patterns of who has been infected. This data is of utmost importance in finding solutions to contain and diminish this severe contagion. In order to produce effective prophylactic and therapeutic strategies, future research needs to understand the sources of severity and complications.

What has been determined is that specific demographics of people seem to have been affected much more than other groups. Certain factors such as individuals with comorbidities (multiple chronic illnesses), specific ethnic backgrounds and older aged people have had a greater risk of contracting the disease. Being obese puts someone more at risk for many serious chronic diseases. Over the last 3 years, obesity is one of the issues that has trended towards making an individual most susceptible to becoming affected by COVID-19 (Mal, et al., 2022).

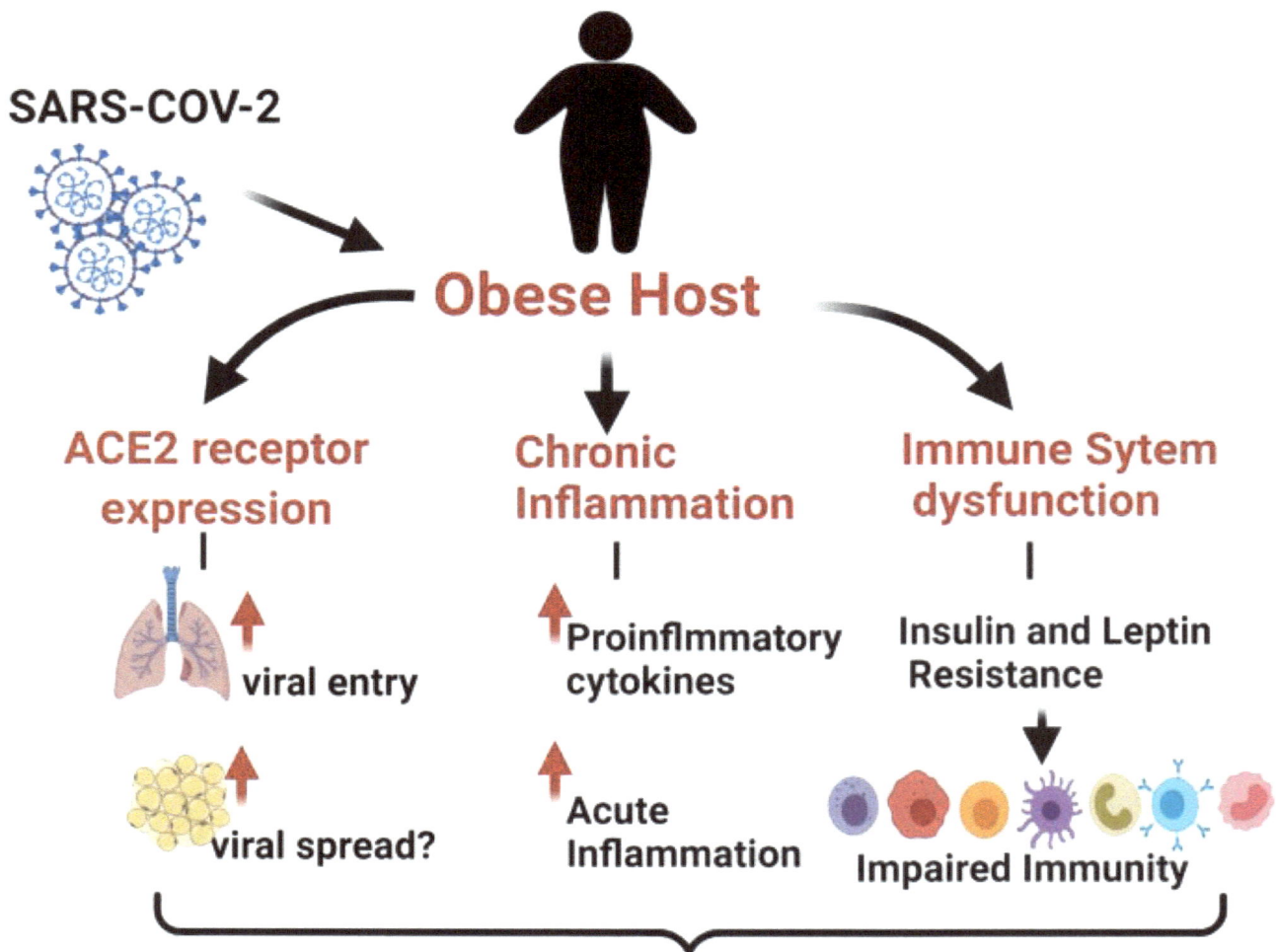

https://immunityageing.biomedcentral.com/articles/10.1186/s12979-020-00212-x

There is much scientific data that supports why biological and physiological mechanisms that fight off disease and illness become compromised due to the various health issues associated with obesity. COVID-19 and its relevance to adiposity are major predictors of severe disease and illness. Hypercytokinemia, immunological, endothelial dysfunction, dysregulation, and cardiovascular impairments are all possible mechanisms, where excess adipose tissue can increase an acute hyper-inflammatory state. This condition is typical of major SARSCoV-2 infections and relative negative symptoms. Increased levels of the pro-inflammatory adipokine leptin, in combination with the anti-inflammatory-acting ACE2 receptors in the lung epithelium of infected individuals, inhibit the innate immune response from being cleared, resulting in a ripple effect of tragic consequences for patients. When adipose tissue and associated immune cells increased cytokine secretion, the immune system can potentially overcompensate as a side-effect of pro-inflammatory "priming," resulting in a cytokine storm. As a consequence of the immune system's inability to produce a sufficient immunological response, virus clearance is compromised. High-risk patients that are at an advance age and/or those with obesity, may be more affected from a less robust immune system response and a lower lasting immunological memory, resulting in limited vaccine effectiveness (Mal, et al., 2022).

The CDC has stated "Hispanic, non-Hispanic Black, and Native American adults have a higher prevalence of obesity and are more likely to suffer worse outcomes from COVID-19. Racial and ethnic minority groups have historically not had broad opportunities for economic, physical, and emotional health, and these inequities have increased the risk of getting sick and dying from COVID-19 for some groups. Many of these same factors are contributing to the higher level of obesity in some racial and ethnic minority groups."

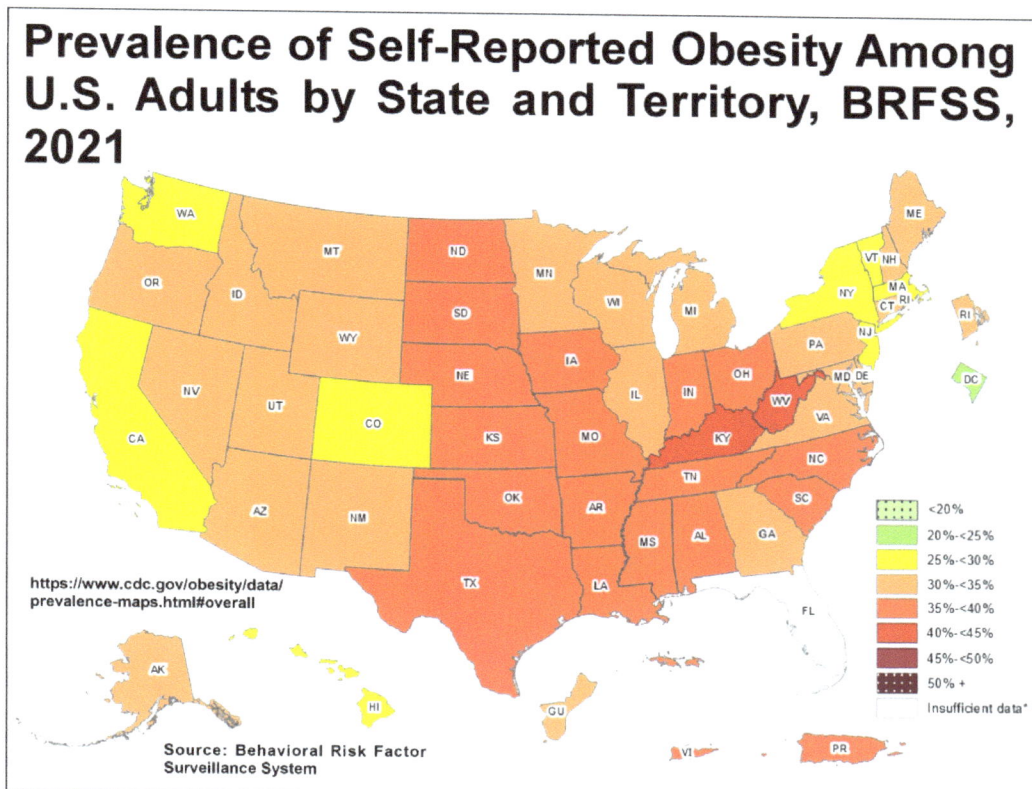

Prevalence of Self-Reported Obesity Among U.S. Adults by State and Territory, BRFSS, 2021

https://www.cdc.gov/obesity/data/prevalence-maps.html#overall

Source: Behavioral Risk Factor Surveillance System

Prevalence of Self-Reported Obesity Among Non-Hispanic American Indian or Alaska Native Adult by State and Territory, BRFSS, 2019–2021

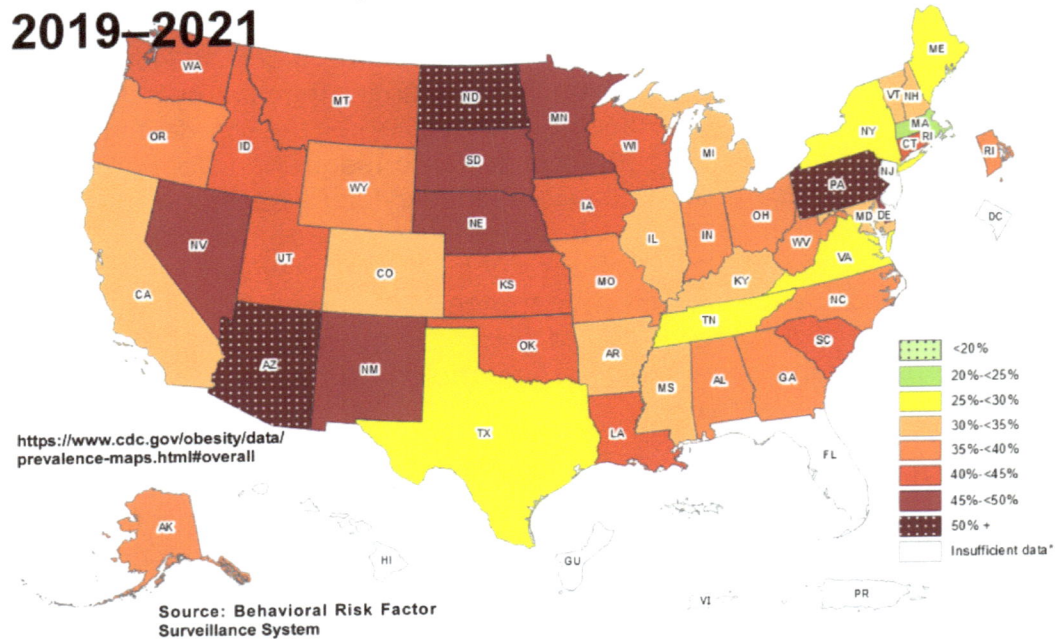

https://www.cdc.gov/obesity/data/prevalence-maps.html#overall

Legend:
- <20%
- 20%-<25%
- 25%-<30%
- 30%-<35%
- 35%-<40%
- 40%-<45%
- 45%-<50%
- 50%+
- Insufficient data*

Source: Behavioral Risk Factor Surveillance System

Prevalence of Self-Reported Obesity Among Hispanic Adults by State and Territory, BRFSS, 2019–2021

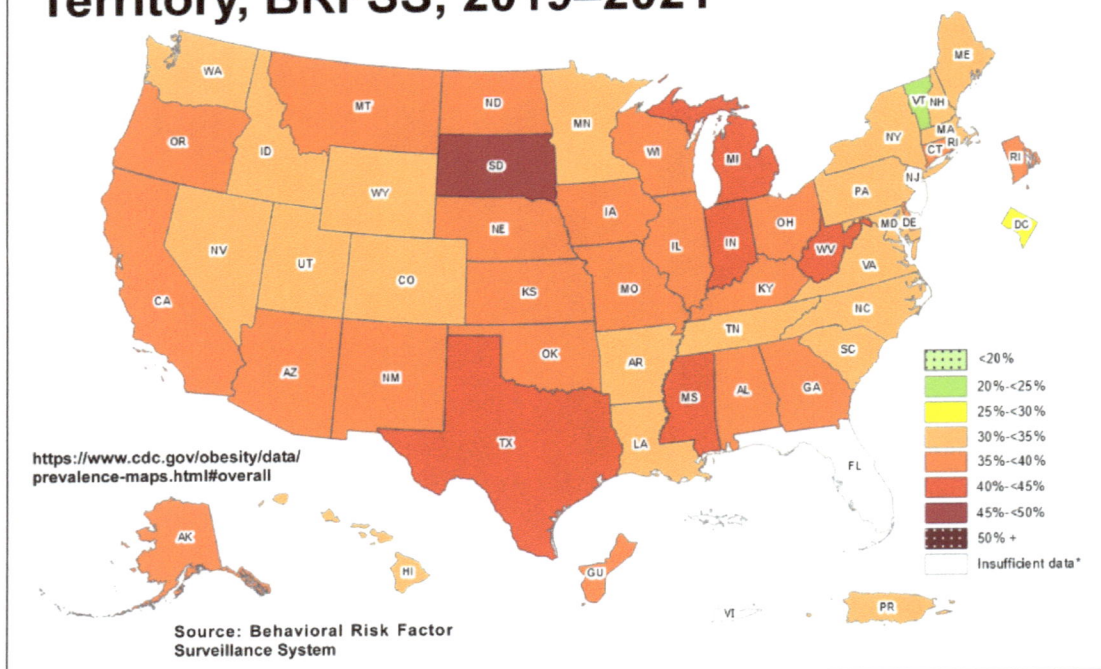

https://www.cdc.gov/obesity/data/prevalence-maps.html#overall

Legend:
- <20%
- 20%-<25%
- 25%-<30%
- 30%-<35%
- 35%-<40%
- 40%-<45%
- 45%-<50%
- 50%+
- Insufficient data*

Source: Behavioral Risk Factor Surveillance System

112

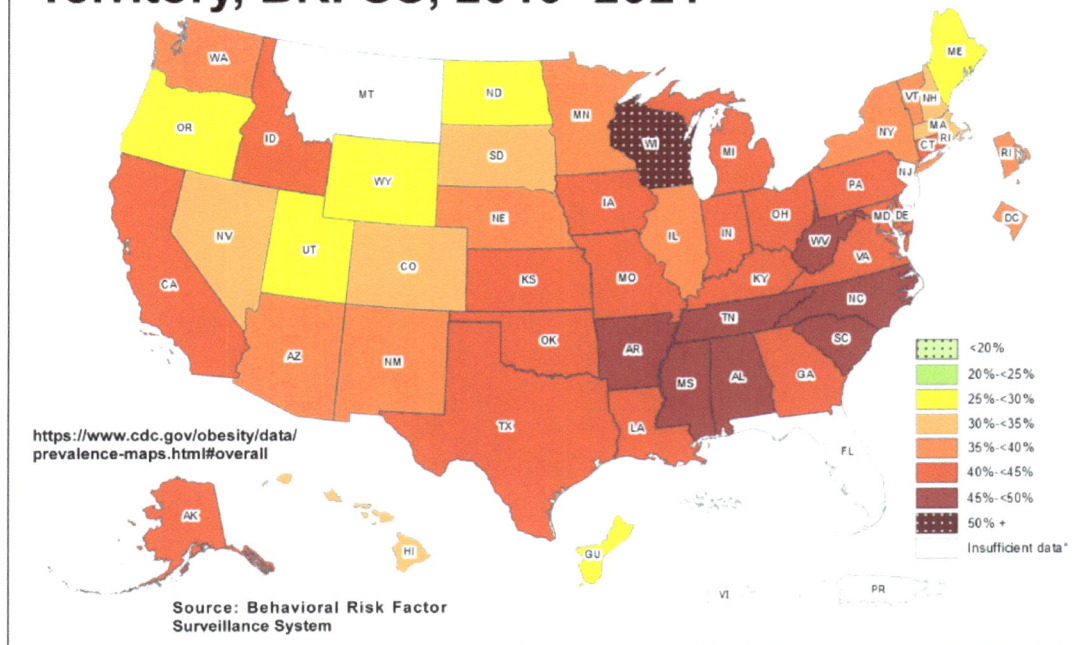

Prevalence of Self-Reported Obesity Among Non-Hispanic Black Adults by State and Territory, BRFSS, 2019–2021

https://www.cdc.gov/obesity/data/prevalence-maps.html#overall

Legend:
- <20%
- 20%-<25%
- 25%-<30%
- 30%-<35%
- 35%-<40%
- 40%-<45%
- 45%-<50%
- 50% +
- Insufficient data*

Source: Behavioral Risk Factor Surveillance System

The pursuit of a healthy lifestyle that can impact on the trajectory of COVID-19 disease, has been one of the most important insights reaped from this catastrophe. Hopefully, this insight will not be squandered until the next public health crisis. Government and political leaders stress that everyone should take action to slow the spread of COVID-19, for the benefit of all.

We seem to have major public health issues occurring every few years. Personal accountability for one's own health, is indeed a way to change our current "sickcare" system to more of a "selfcare" system where people don't wait to become sick before adopting a healthy lifestyle.

Systemic change does not happen overnight. Long-term weight loss is a work in progress. Some immediate steps that individuals can take to help protect themselves as well as their families during a pandemic are:

- Eat a healthy diet
- Use supplements as necessary and not as a substitute
- Become more active
- Execute regular physical activity
- Get adequate sleep

- Learn how to cope better with stress

- Get adequate sun exposure to promote vitamin D production and natural immunity

These actions can help most individuals with obesity by improving their overall health. These actions can help to lower blood pressure, lower blood cholesterol, and lower blood sugars. With a lower body mass index or BMI, the risk of severe illnesses contributing to contracting COVID-19, as well as many other common diseases and illness can be reduced.

References:

https://www.cdc.gov/obesity/data/obesity-and-covid-19.html

Mal, P., Mukherjee, T., Upadhyay, A. K., Mohanty, S., & Pattnaik, A. K. (2022). Connecting the dots between inflammatory cascades of obesity and COVID-19 in light of mortal consequences-a review. Environmental science and pollution research international, 29(38), 57040–57053. https://doi.org/10.1007/s11356-022-21461-x

Mohammad, S., Aziz, R., Al Mahri, S. *et al.* Obesity and COVID-19: what makes obese host so vulnerable?. *Immun Ageing* **18**, 1 (2021). https://doi.org/10.1186/s12979-020-00212-x

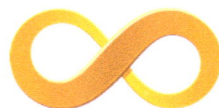

SECTION V: STRESS, CIRCULATION, & EMOTIONAL HEALTH

How do you deal with stress?

- take a few deep breaths
- drink a few alcoholic beverages
- take pharmaceuticals
- consume some form of Marijuana, hallucinogen, or psychedelic
- physical exercise
- listen to soothing music
- do nothing

In order to better manage stress, wouldn't it help to better understand what stress is, and how it affects our bodies physiologically? Do we truly manage our stressors or just go with the "band-aid" approach of treating symptoms rather than addressing root causes?

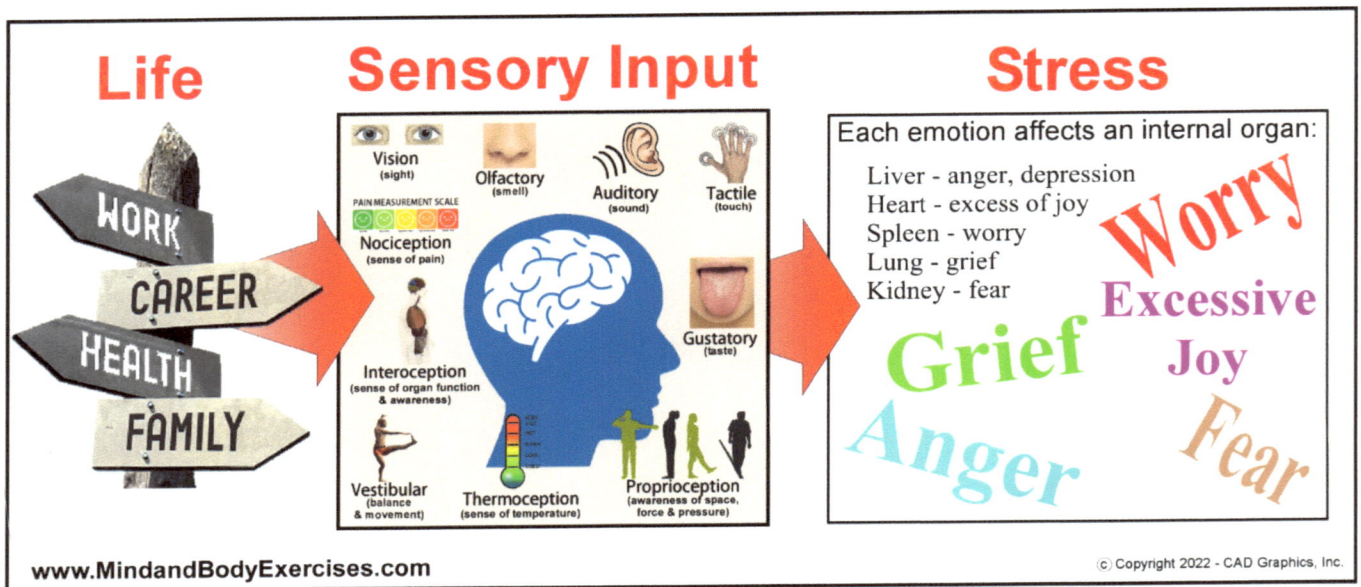

Life and the experiences that it offers is constantly changing and evolving for all that exist. Our senses are continuously receiving and interpreting stimulus to determine what is good or bad for our survival. Consequently, this input often manifests into what we call stress. We deal with stress through our thoughts and emotions. Our emotions directly affect how our brain processes information that affects all of our physiological mechanism and organ functions through the autonomic nervous and endocrine systems. Basically, thoughts and emotions affect our health and well-being whether with positive or negative outcomes.

The HPA-axis
(Hypothalamus-Pituitary-Adrenal)
How the Stress Response Works

The HPA-Axis is the physiological mechanism for how the mind and body respond to stress.

1 – Receptors sense stress stimuli and send chemical signals to the hypothalamus, which releases corticotropic (CRH) to the pituitary gland. The pituitary gland then releases adrenocorticotropic (ACTH) to the adrenal glands.

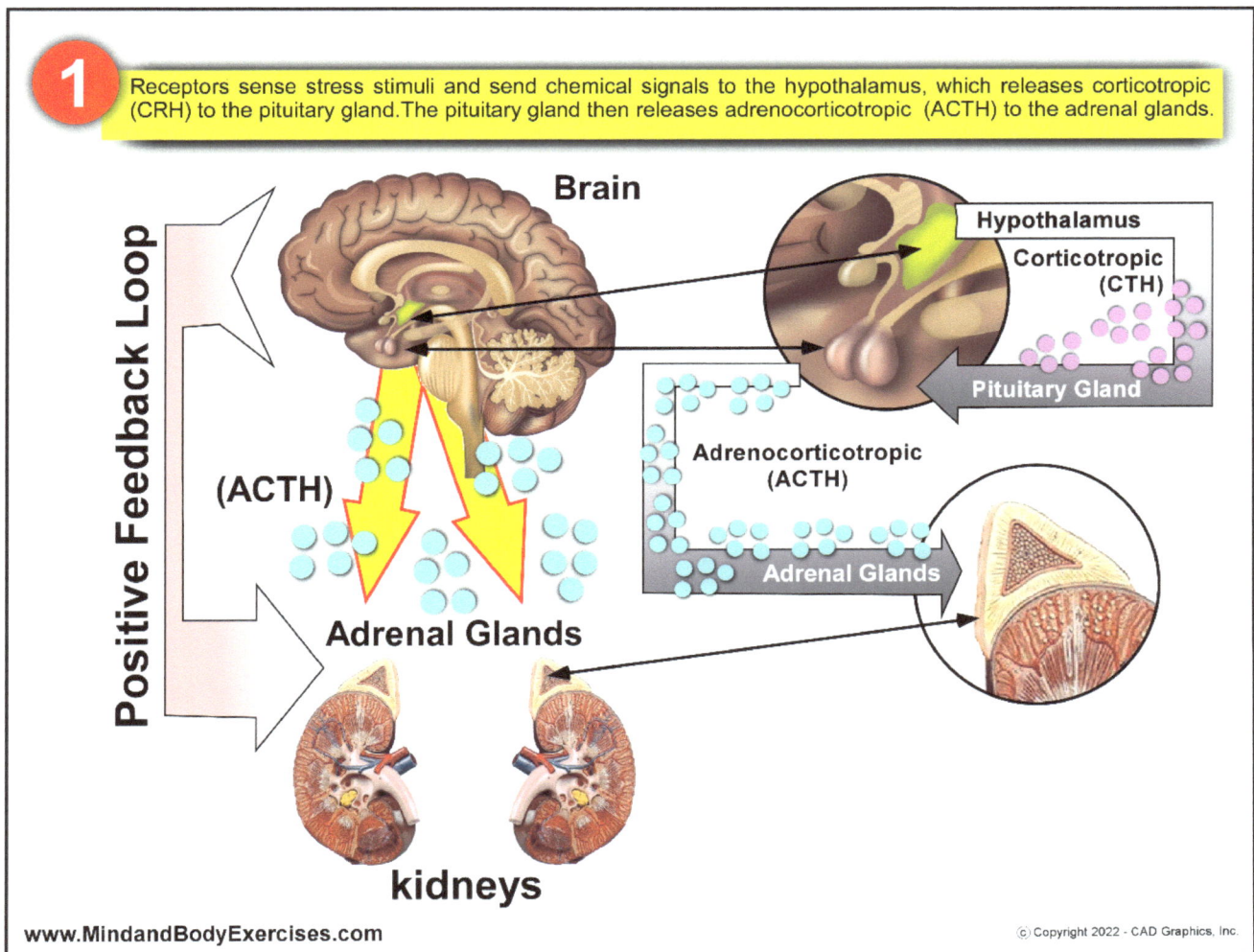

1 Receptors sense stress stimuli and send chemical signals to the hypothalamus, which releases corticotropic (CRH) to the pituitary gland.The pituitary gland then releases adrenocorticotropic (ACTH) to the adrenal glands.

Brain

Positive Feedback Loop

(ACTH)

Hypothalamus

Corticotropic (CTH)

Pituitary Gland

Adrenocorticotropic (ACTH)

Adrenal Glands

Adrenal Glands

kidneys

2 – The adrenal glands respond with the secretion of cortisol, adrenaline, and noradrenaline to be released into the bloodstream.

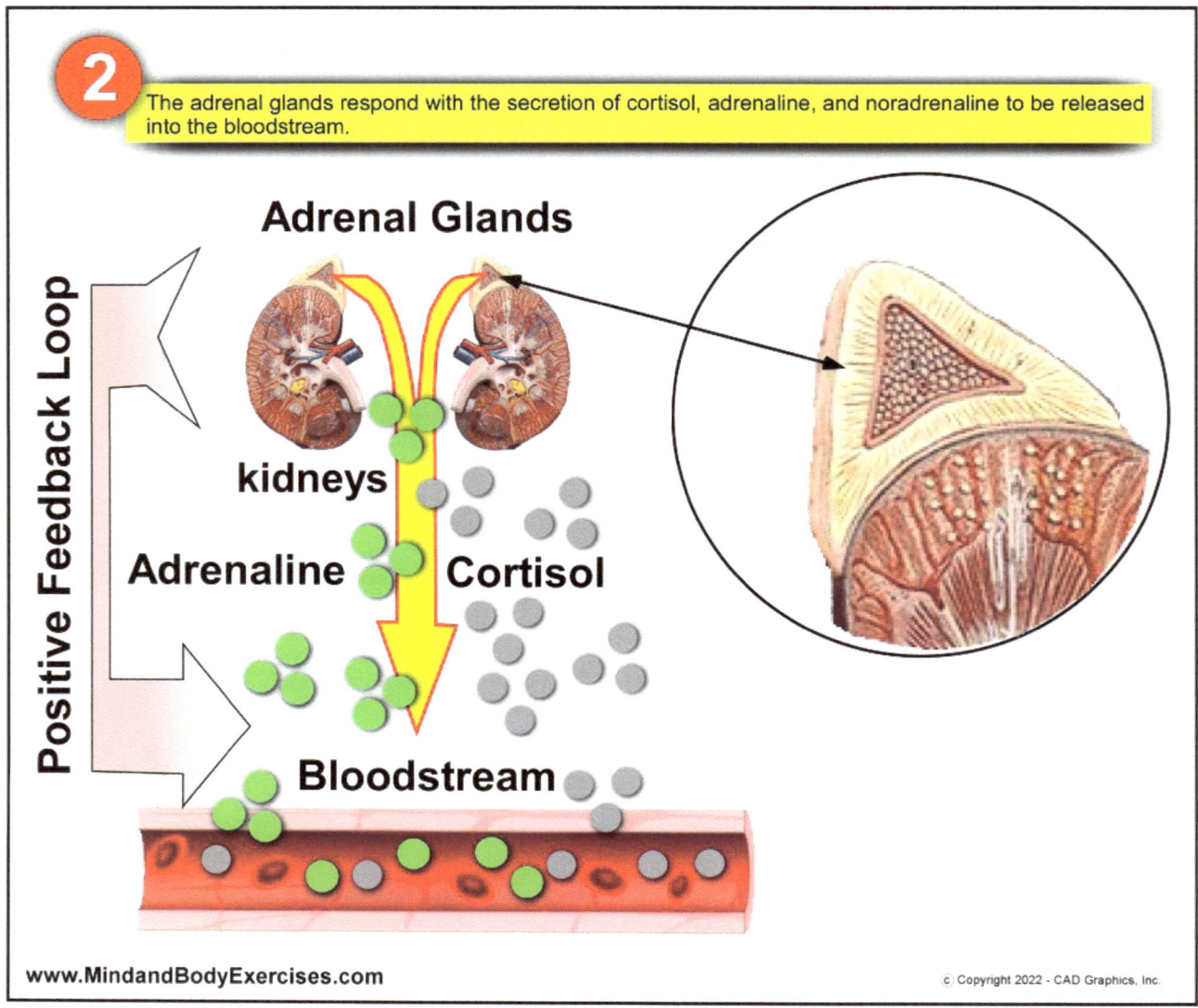

2 The adrenal glands respond with the secretion of cortisol, adrenaline, and noradrenaline to be released into the bloodstream.

Adrenal Glands

Positive Feedback Loop

kidneys

Adrenaline   **Cortisol**

Bloodstream

3 – Immediate physiological changes are induced, including acceleration of heart and lung activity, elevated blood pressure, inhibition of digestive activity, tunnel vision, and sweating. Cortisol levels are then reported back to the hypothalamus, completing a negative feedback loop to repeat the whole process as necessary.

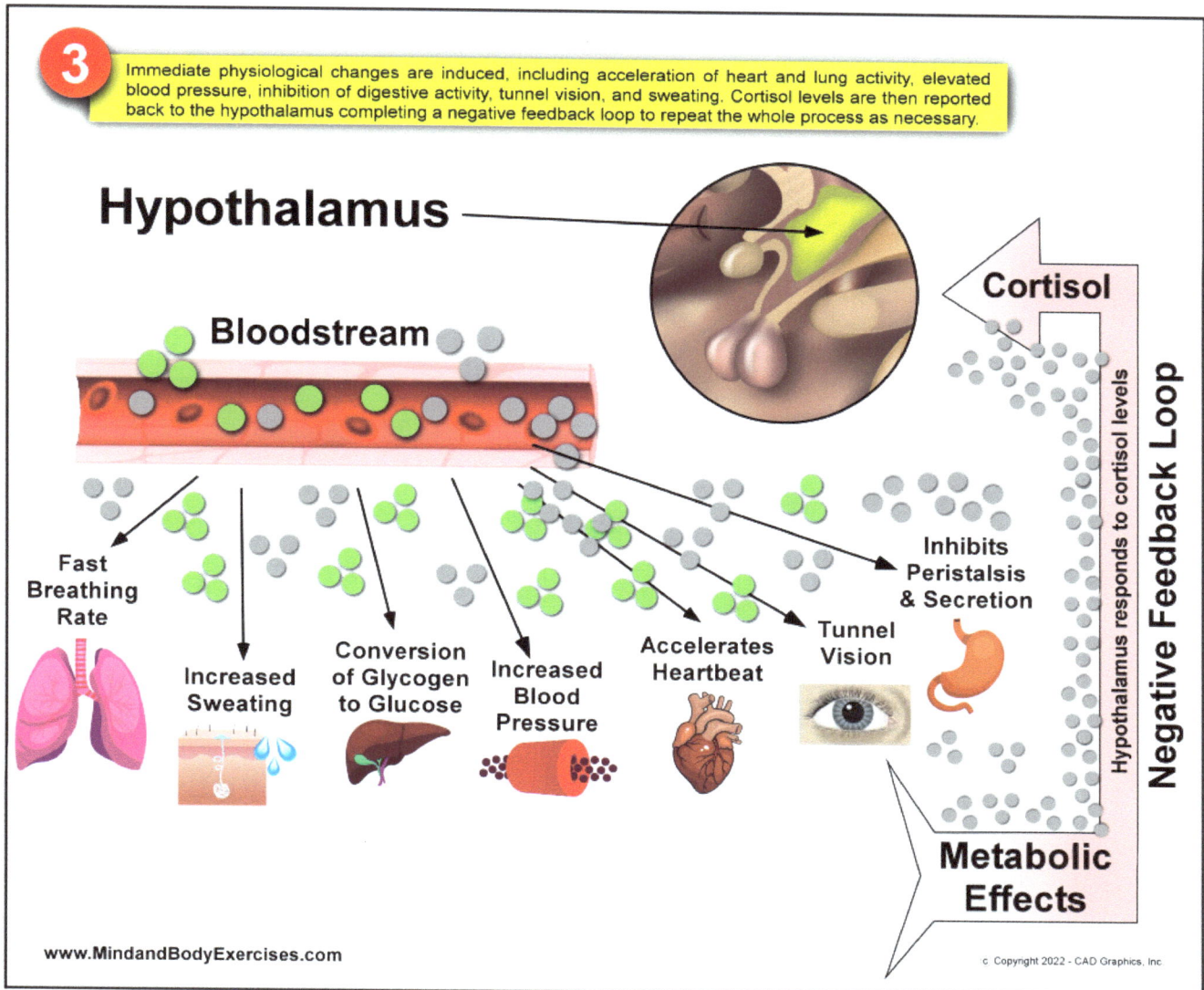

3 Immediate physiological changes are induced, including acceleration of heart and lung activity, elevated blood pressure, inhibition of digestive activity, tunnel vision, and sweating. Cortisol levels are then reported back to the hypothalamus completing a negative feedback loop to repeat the whole process as necessary.

Why is this important to understand? Because when cortisol levels are too high for prolonged periods of time, other physiological mechanisms become impaired. When levels are balanced cortisol plays in important role in regulating blood chemistry:

- Increases gluconeogenesis
- Mobilizes fatty acids from adipose
- Break down stored proteins
- Enhances SNS response
- Puts brakes on inflammation/immune response

Negative effects would include:

- Increased insulin resistance
- Altered perception & emotion in the central nervous system
- Suppressed GH release
- Suppressed TSH and inhibits peripheral activation of T4 into T3
- Inhibited bone remodeling
- Suppressed reproductive function

We do have the ability to consciously control and manage our stress whether through lifestyle choices, diet & nutrition, physical activity and attitude. A key component of managing stress is managing the parasympathetic (rest & digest) and sympathetic (fight or flight) nervous system through consistent regulation of our breathing frequency and relative volume of each breath. This is a topic addressed in many of my other posts. Yoga, tai chi, qigong, meditation, martial arts and other methods have been proven to help to proactively manage stress and relative cortisol levels.

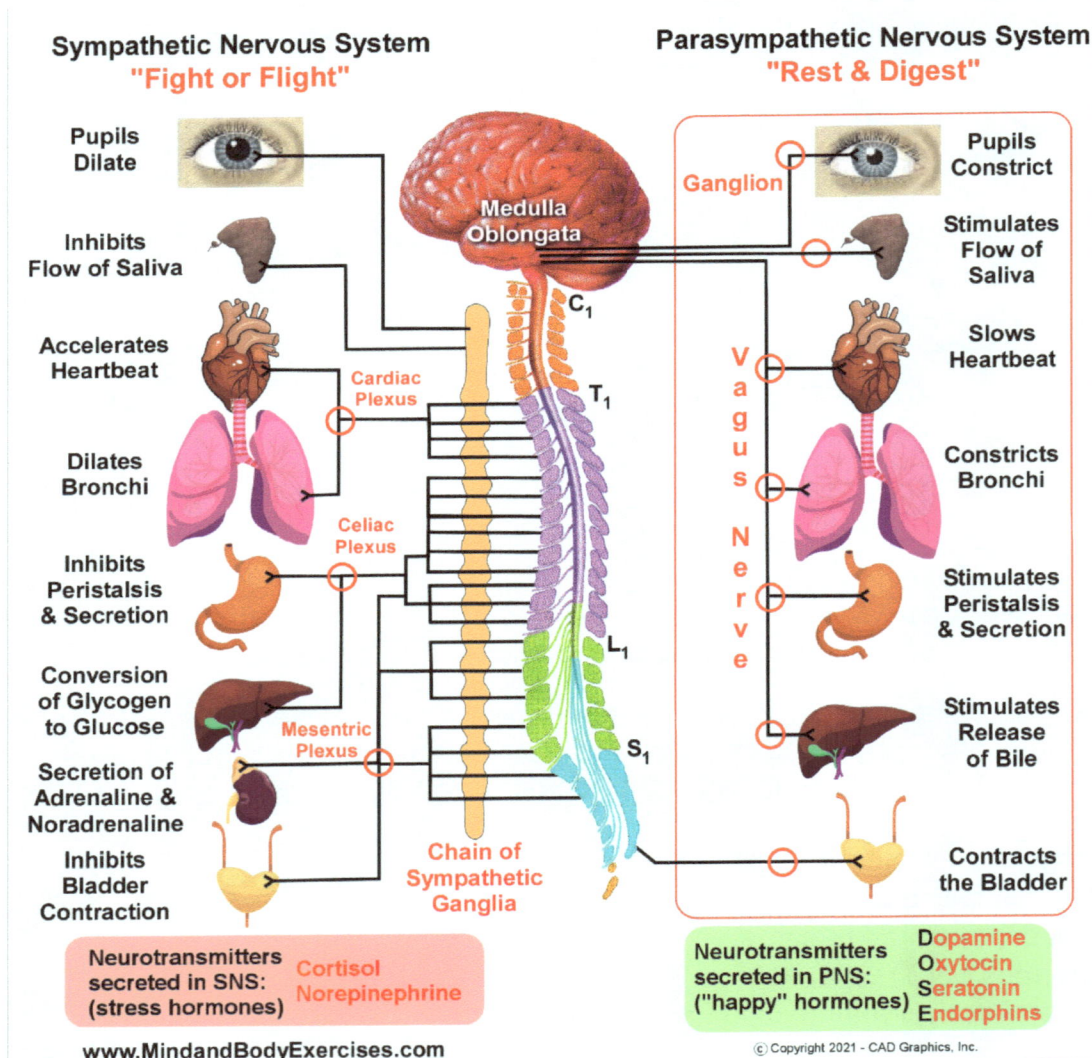

Life

Sensory Input

Stress

WORK
CAREER
HEALTH
FAMILY

Vision (sight)
Olfactory (smell)
Auditory (sound)
Tactile (touch)

PAIN MEASUREMENT SCALE

Nociception (sense of pain)

Interoception (sense of organ function & awareness)

Gustatory (taste)

Vestibular (balance & movement)
Thermoception (sense of temperature)
Proprioception (awareness of space, force and pressure)

Each emotion affects an internal organ:

Liver - anger, depression
Heart - excess of joy
Spleen - worry
Lung - grief
Kidney - fear

Worry

Excessive Joy

Grief

Anger

Fear

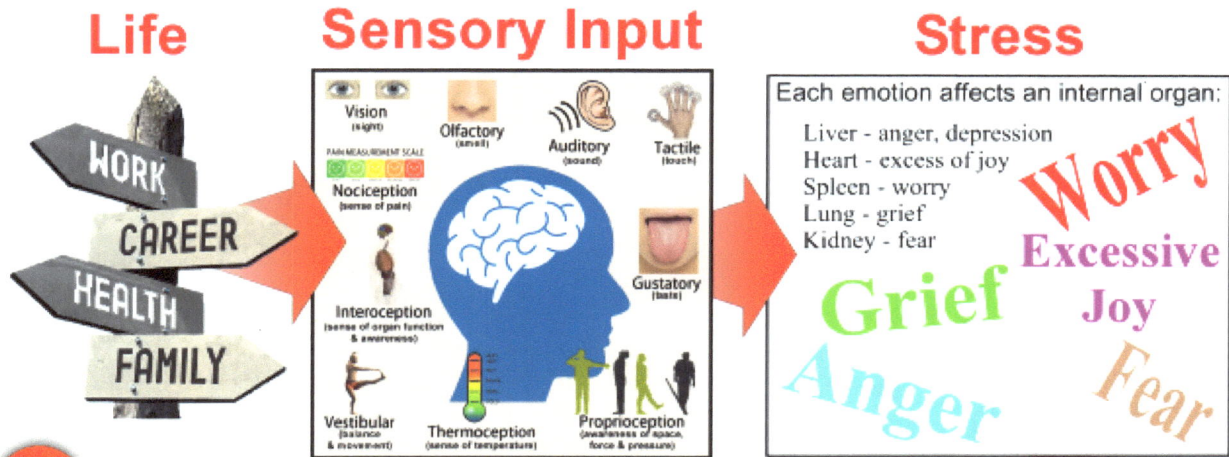

1 Receptors sense stress stimuli and send chemical signals to the hypothalamus, which releases corticotropic (CRH) to the pituitary gland. The pituitary gland then releases adrenocorticotropic (ACTH) to the adrenal glands.

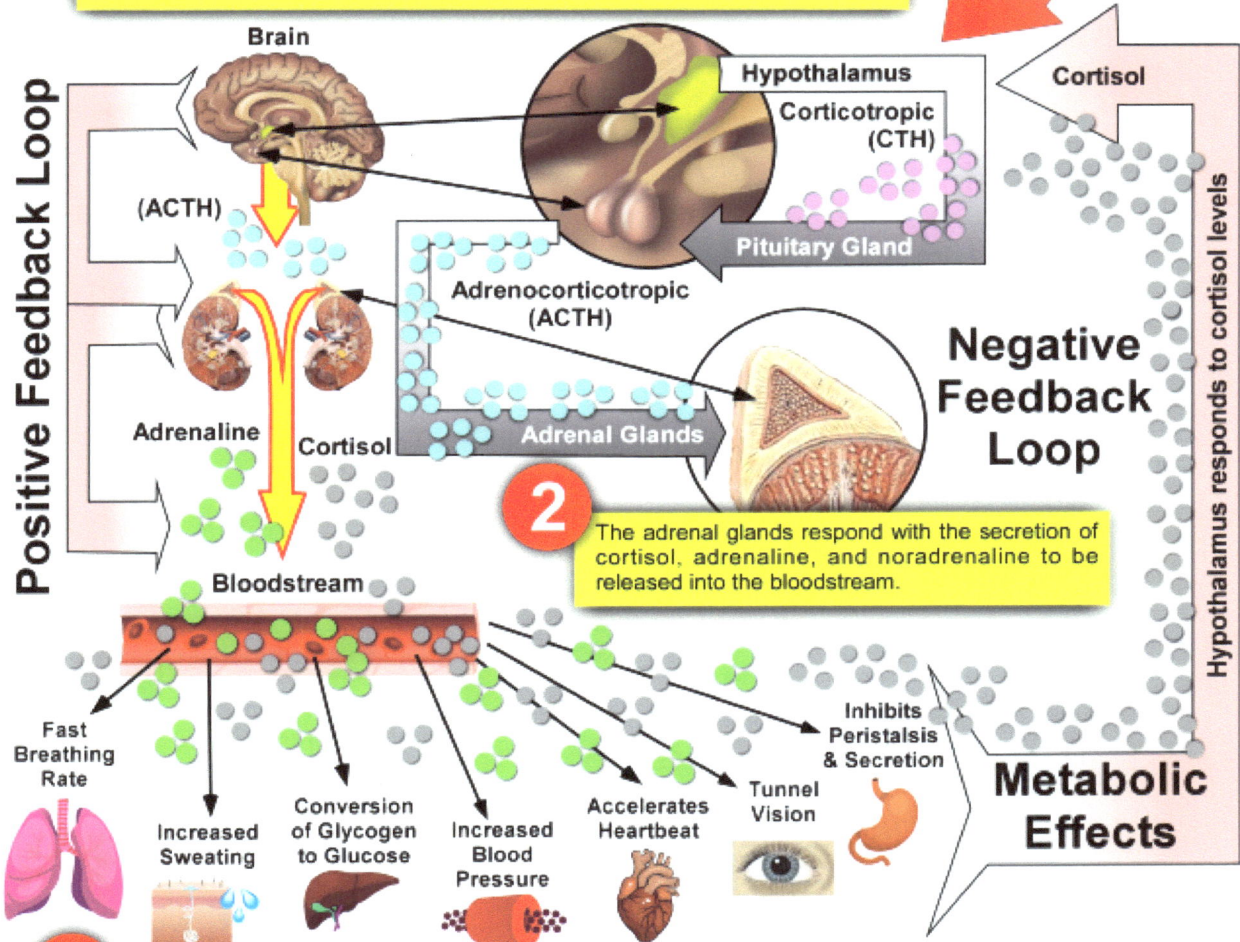

Positive Feedback Loop

Brain

(ACTH)

Adrenaline

Cortisol

Bloodstream

Hypothalamus
Corticotropic (CTH)

Pituitary Gland

Adrenocorticotropic (ACTH)

Cortisol

Negative Feedback Loop

Adrenal Glands

Hypothalamus responds to cortisol levels

2 The adrenal glands respond with the secretion of cortisol, adrenaline, and noradrenaline to be released into the bloodstream.

Fast Breathing Rate

Increased Sweating

Conversion of Glycogen to Glucose

Increased Blood Pressure

Accelerates Heartbeat

Tunnel Vision

Inhibits Peristalsis & Secretion

Metabolic Effects

3 Immediate physiological changes are induced, including acceleration of heart and lung activity, elevated blood pressure, inhibition of digestive activity, tunnel vision, and sweating.

Acupressure (no needles) and its parent of acupuncture (needles) from Traditional Chinese medicine, has been around for a few thousand years.

An Acupuncture Mechanism Theory

1 Pain manifests where a fascial triad (veins, arteries and nerves) is choked by collagen.

2 Free endings of veins, arteries and nerves (fascial triad) are roughly 82% identical to the 361 acupoints on the human body.

3 Needle is inserted at acupoints and then manipulated by twisting the needle thereby deforming the collagen of the fascia.

4 Choked collagen is deformed by the acupuncture needle, causing piezoelectric forces or pressure signals to be relayed via neural network.

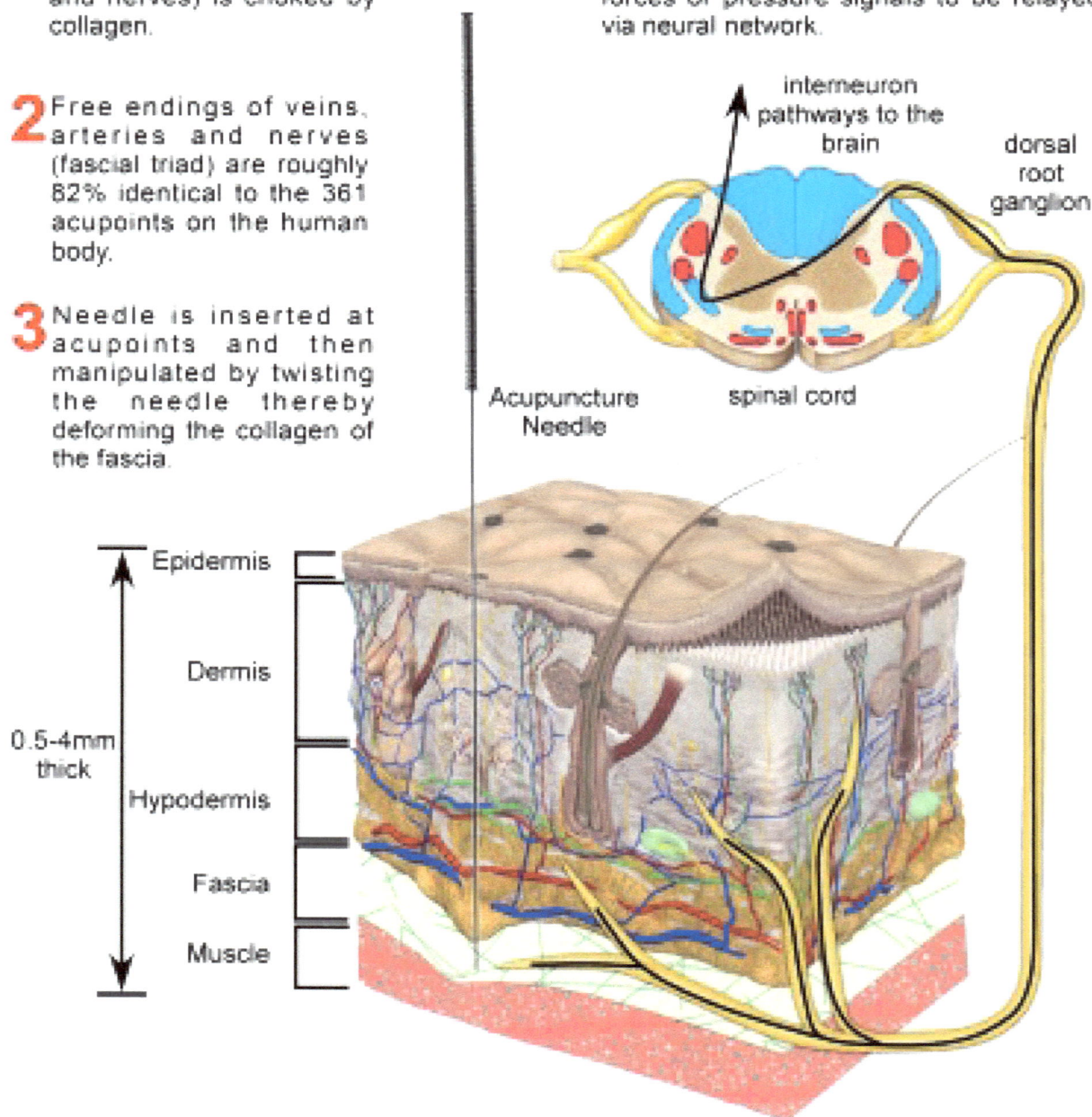

interneuron pathways to the brain

dorsal root ganglion

spinal cord

Acupuncture Needle

Epidermis

Dermis

0.5-4mm thick

Hypodermis

Fascia

Muscle

An Acupuncture Mechanism Theory (con't.)

5 Unchoking of the collagen releases endorphins such as Substance P (SP) within the spinal column to block pain perception and provide relief.

6 Substance P is released by nerves that bind with mast cells.

7 Mast cells produce receptors for Substance P binding.

8 Histamine, Heparin & Neurokinin-A are release by mast cells.

9 Electric sensation is felt.

10 Action potential travels through nerves activating signal to the brain.

11 Signals reach the hypothalamus & pituitary glands affecting the autonomic nervous system and consequently blood pressure, healing response and other bodily functions.

12 The insula cortex of the brain maintains homeostasis by regulating sympathetic and parasympathetic response of the internal organs

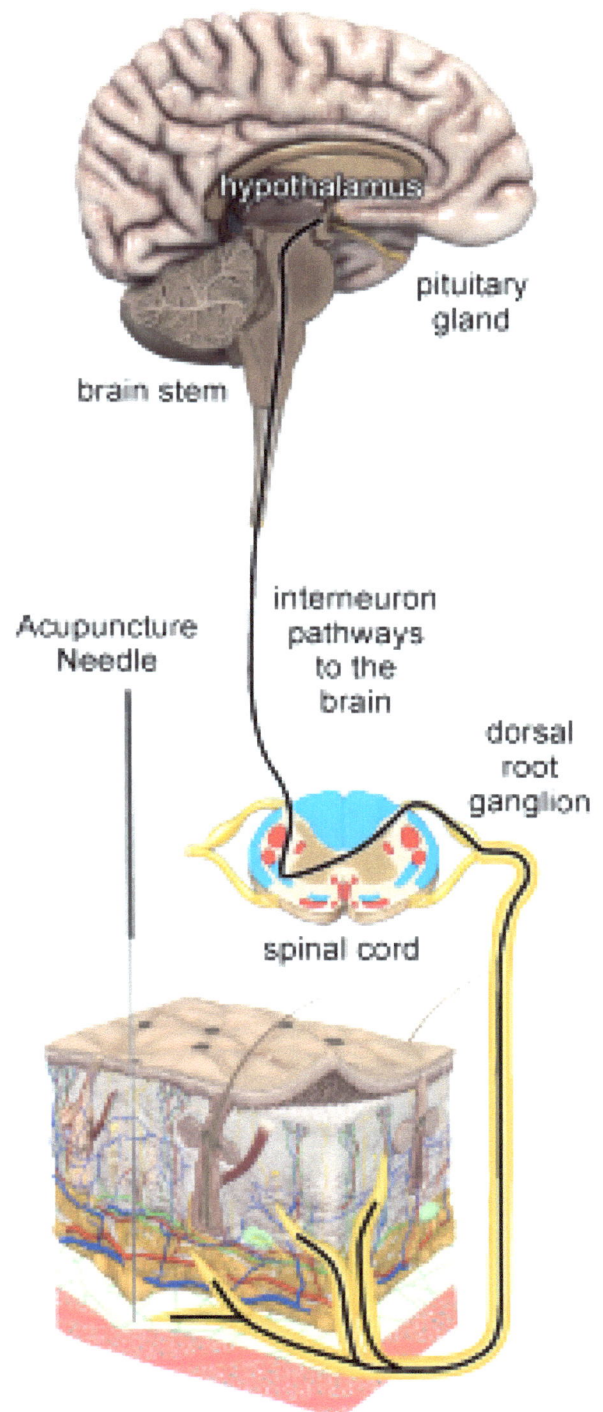

hypothalamus

pituitary gland

brain stem

interneuron pathways to the brain

Acupuncture Needle

dorsal root ganglion

spinal cord

There is an amazing amount of knowledge, methods and alternative options to manage chronic pain beyond surgery, opiates and anti-inflammatories.

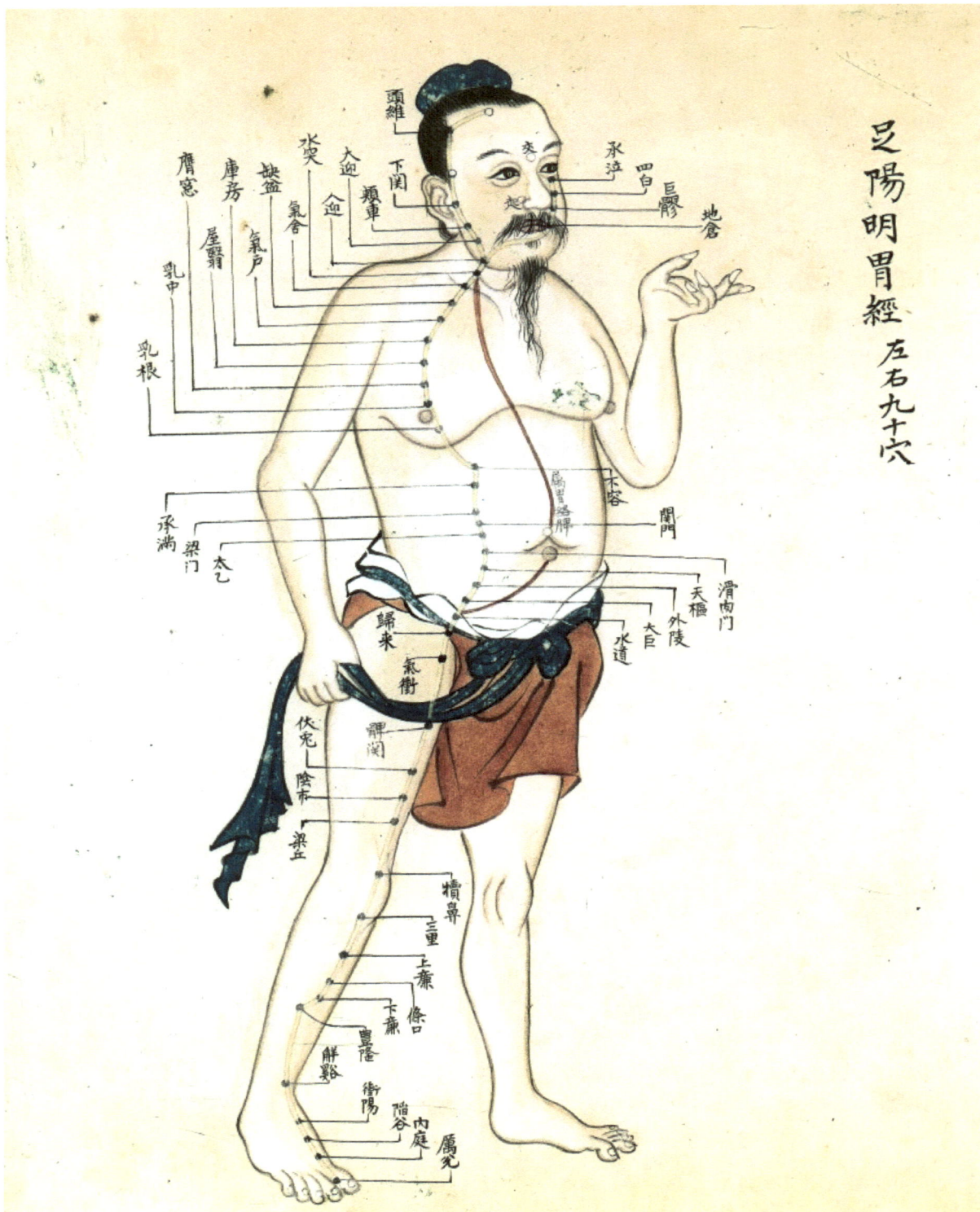

These are techniques that I was taught over 40 years ago from my martial arts masters and teachers. The key factor is consistency – practicing the techniques on a regular basis can help relieve the chronic pain associated with headaches and the stress that often accompanies these issues.

Acupressure - Same concept but no needles!

Similar to acupuncture but using direct pressure to stimulate energy flow within the energy meridians. Acupressure is also the same as reflexology, which is mostly massaging the acupoints on the hands and feet. Acupressure points are located throughout the whole body, allowing for many more points of treatment. The auricle (outer ear) is a micro system, which reflects the entire body and its individual components. Acupuncture & acupressure methods can be applied to the ear acupoints.

Foot Reflexology

Auricular Therapy

Headache & Stress
Acupoints

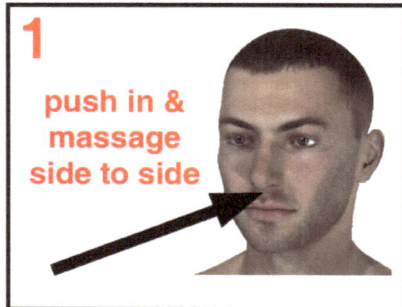

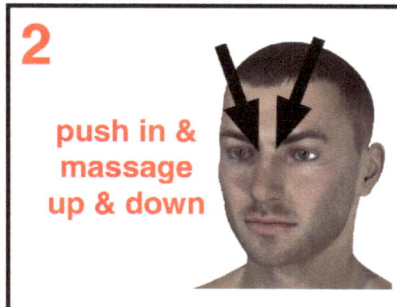

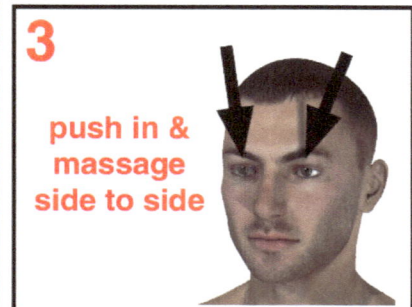

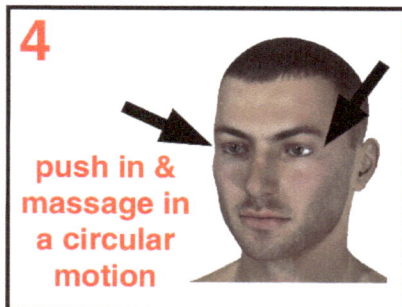

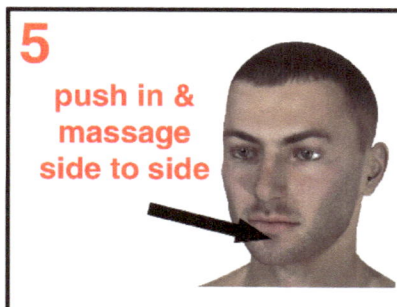

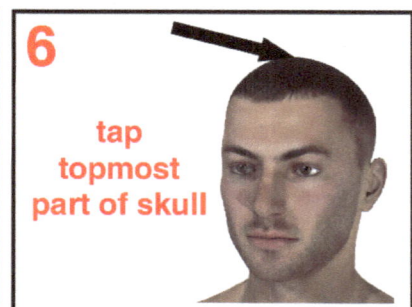

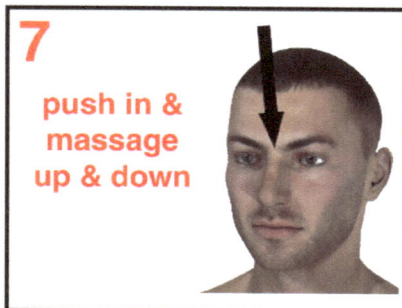

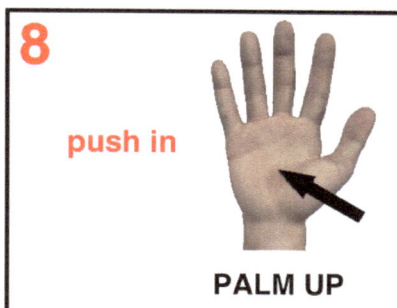

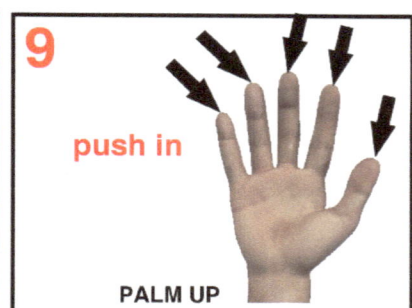

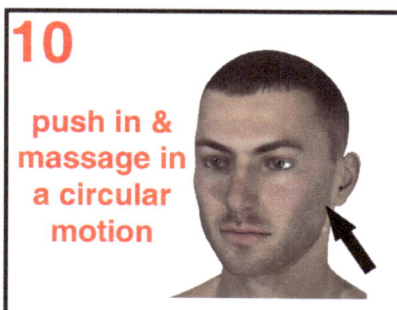

1 push in & massage side to side

2 push in & massage up & down

3 push in & massage side to side

4 push in & massage in a circular motion

5 push in & massage side to side

6 tap topmost part of skull

7 push in & massage up & down

8 push in — PALM UP

9 push in — PALM UP

10 push in & massage in a circular motion

It is easy to see how the time of the day affects us. If you pay attention to it you will see the pattern. During a 24-hour period, our body, energy and emotions change. Knowing this pattern makes daily life much easier. This pattern is known as the Horary Cycle or Circadian Rhythm.

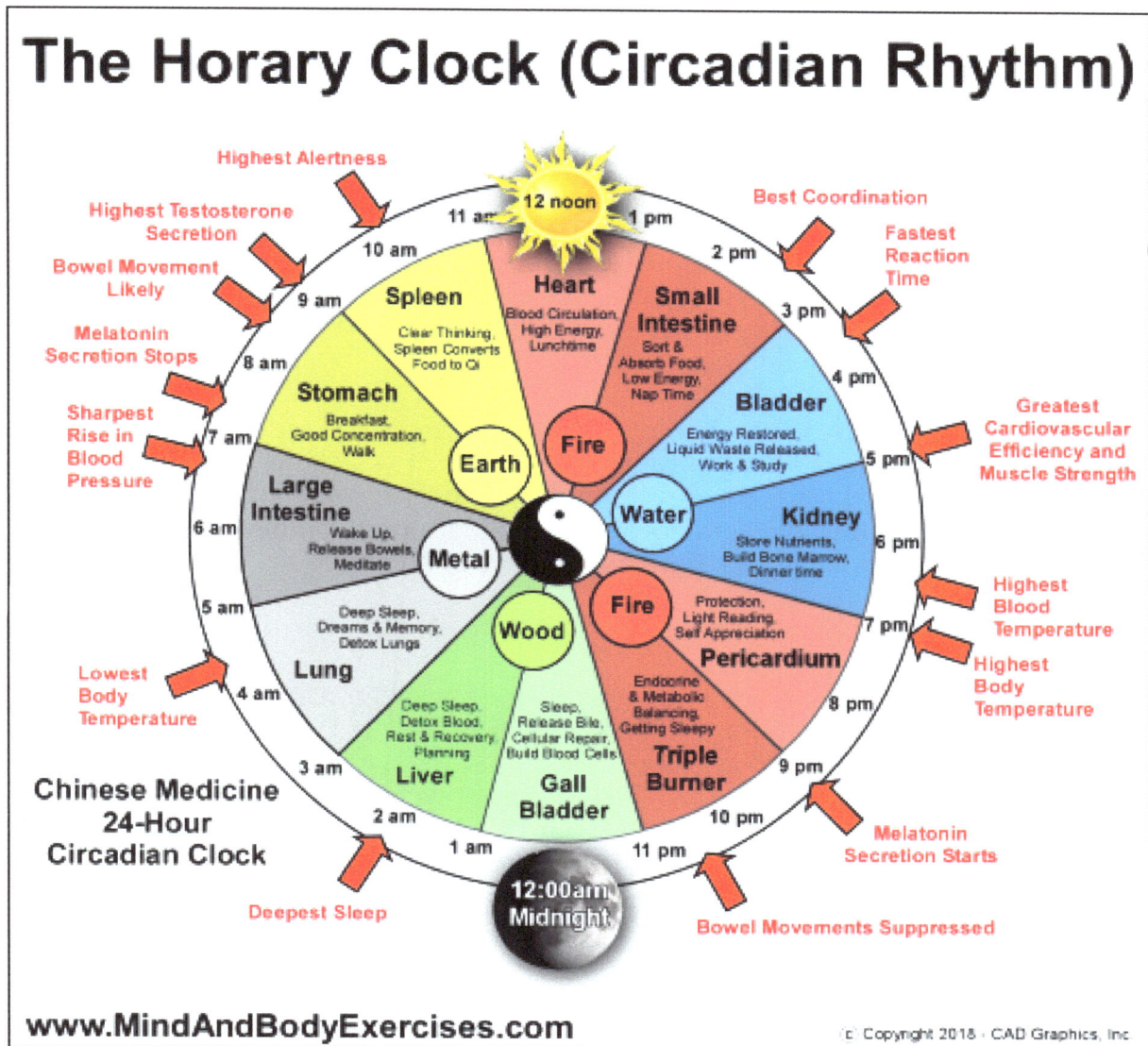

Harmonizing our habits with this cycle would look something like this… From 5-7am, the large intestine is most active. This is the time of the sharpest rise in blood pressure. It's best to take a few deep breaths before rising out of bed. Once out of bed, evacuate our bowels and sit to meditate. From 7-9am, the stomach is most active. The melatonin secretion stops. This is a good time to eat breakfast, take a walk and digest the morning's meal. From 9-11am, the spleen is most active. Highest testosterone secretion of the day. This is the best time for concentration and planning. By starting our day with this schedule, we would maximize both our time and productivity.

Between the hours of 11am and 1pm, the heart is most active. The body is at its most coordinated by noon. This is the best time to exercise, work and to eat our main meal. From 1-3pm, the small intestine is active. This is a low energy time of the day. Absorbing nutrients, short naps and work is best. From 3-5pm, the bladder is most active. This is the fastest reaction time of the day. Walking, working and studying are most beneficial. The kidneys are most active between 5-7pm. This is when we enjoy the greatest cardiovascular efficiency and muscle strength, the highest blood temperature and highest body temperature. Exercise, outdoor activities and a light meal is best. This schedule would regulate the energy throughout the day.

The evening should be reserved for rejuvenation and recovery from the day's activities. From 7-9pm, the pericardium or 'master of the heart' is active. Light reading, massaging the feet and body. The Triple Burner or Triple Heater is at high tide from 9-11pm. The body begins to release melatonin and suppresses bowel movement. Calm socializing and relaxing with friends and family is best.

It is best to be fast asleep by 11pm. From 11pm to 1am, the gall bladder is most active. Releasing bile, cellular repair and blood cell renewal. From 1-3 am, the liver is most active. Deep sleep and liver/blood detox begins. From 3-5 am the lungs are most active. Deep sleep, dreams and lung detox. This is when most people tend to snore the most. Keeping to this schedule would ensure optimal health of the mind, body and spirit.

The Horary Clock (Circadian Rhythm) – 24 Hour Qi Flow Though the Meridians

Understanding how the human body works and interacts within nature, along with self-awareness are the basis of Traditional Chinese medicine.

The graphics ahead show what is known as the Horary cycle or the Circadian Clock. As Qi (energy) makes its way through the meridians, each meridian in turn with its associated organ, has a two-hour period during which it is at maximum energy. The Horary Effect is recognizable by measurable increases of Qi within an organ system and meridian during its time of maximum energy.

Harmonizing Habits:

5-7am – Wake Up, Move Bowels, Meditate
7-9am – Sex, Breakfast, Walk, Digest
9-11am – Work, Best Concentration
11am-1pm – Eat Main Meal of Day, Walk
1-3pm – Absorb Food, Short Nap, Work
3-5pm – Work or Study

5-7pm – Exercise, Light Dinner
7-9pm – Light Reading, Massage Feet
9-11pm – Calm Socializing, Flirting, Sex
11pm-1am – Go to Sleep, Cellular Repair
1-3am – Deep Sleep, Detox Liver & Blood
3-5am – Deep Sleep, Detox Lungs

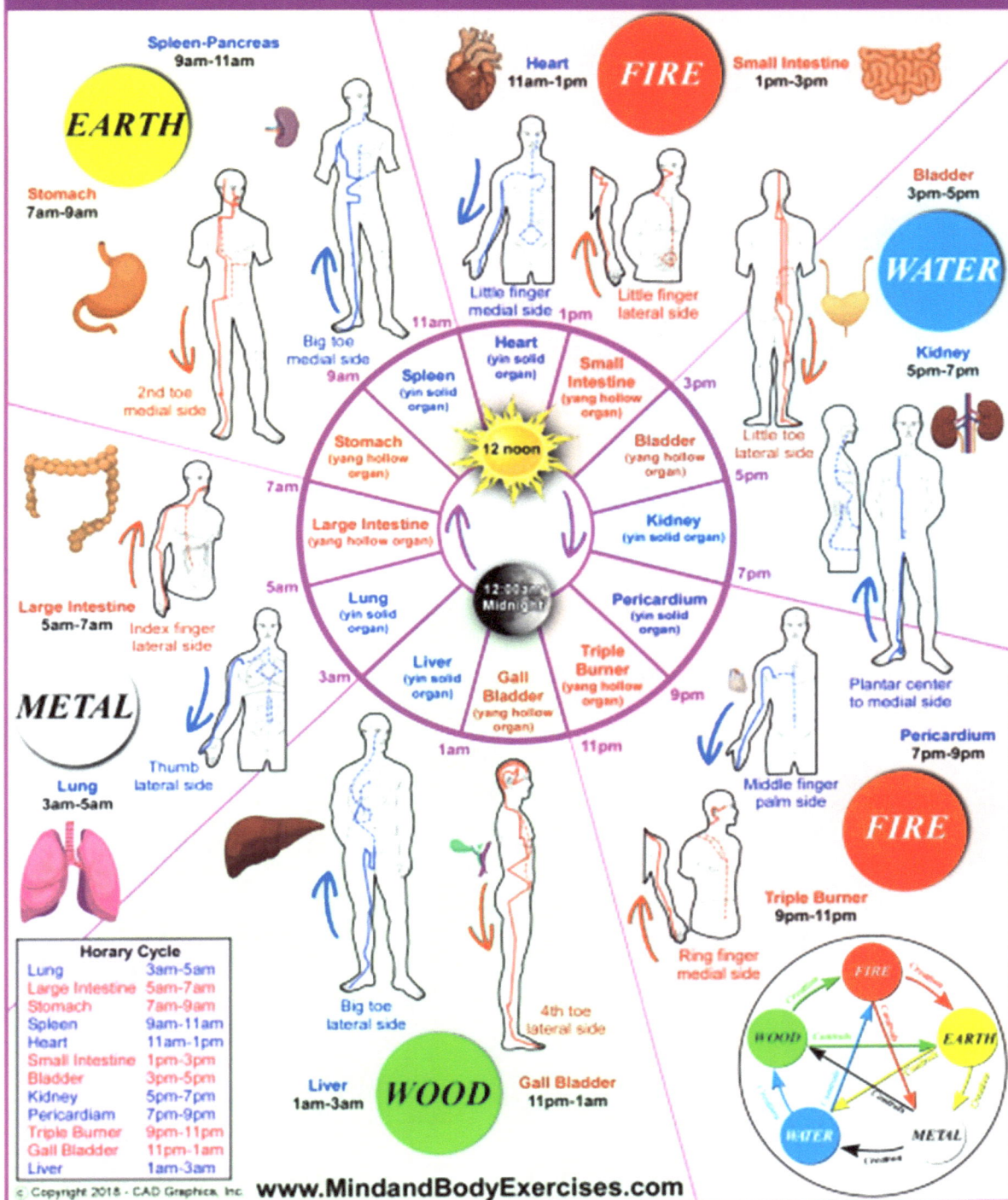

Daily Energy Flow in the 12 Main Meridians & Related Organs

Spleen-Pancreas 9am-11am

EARTH

Stomach 7am-9am

2nd toe medial side

Big toe medial side 9am

11am

Heart 11am-1pm

FIRE

Small Intestine 1pm-3pm

Little finger medial side

Little finger lateral side 1pm

Bladder 3pm-5pm

WATER

Kidney 5pm-7pm

Little toe lateral side 3pm

Large Intestine 5am-7am

Index finger lateral side

METAL

Lung 3am-5am

Thumb lateral side 5am

7pm

5pm

Plantar center to medial side

Pericardium 7pm-9pm

FIRE

Triple Burner 9pm-11pm

Ring finger medial side

Middle finger palm side

Central Wheel:
- Spleen (yin solid organ)
- Stomach (yang hollow organ)
- Large Intestine (yang hollow organ)
- Lung (yin solid organ)
- Liver (yin solid organ)
- Gall Bladder (yang hollow organ)
- Triple Burner (yang hollow organ)
- Pericardium (yin solid organ)
- Kidney (yin solid organ)
- Bladder (yang hollow organ)
- Small Intestine (yang hollow organ)
- Heart (yin solid organ)

12 noon — 12:00 Midnight

7am — 5am — 3am — 1am — 11pm — 9pm

Big toe lateral side

4th toe lateral side

Liver 1am-3am

WOOD

Gall Bladder 11pm-1am

Horary Cycle

Lung	3am-5am
Large Intestine	5am-7am
Stomach	7am-9am
Spleen	9am-11am
Heart	11am-1pm
Small Intestine	1pm-3pm
Bladder	3pm-5pm
Kidney	5pm-7pm
Pericardiam	7pm-9pm
Triple Burner	9pm-11pm
Gall Bladder	11pm-1am
Liver	1am-3am

www.MindandBodyExercises.com

FIRE — WOOD — EARTH — WATER — METAL

114

Setting the 24-hour circadian rhythm

Environment/daily patterns (eating/sleeping/exercising)

Genes

Day

Night

Go to sleep

Change length of day to match seasons

Melatonin

Daylight = off
Night-time = on

SCN +

PinG

Serotonin

PIT

Raphe

'MASTER CLOCK' SCN = suprachiasmatic nucleus (in the hypothalamus – sets the time)
PIT = pituitary gland
PinG = pineal gland
ACTH = adrenocorticotropic hormone
TSH = thyroid-stimulating hormone

Key stimulating hormones

ACTH   TSH   Autonomic nervous system   Body temperature

ORGAN LEVEL

Adrenal gland	Thyroid gland	Heart	Pancreas	Liver	Fat	Muscle	Gut
cortisol	thyroid hormone		insulin	glycogen	lipid metabolism		

Food and activity

DAY

Muscle
• Fatty acid uptake
• Glycolitic metabolism

Fat
• Lipogenesis
• Adiponectin production

Liver
• Glycogen synthesis
• Cholesterol synthesis
• Bile acid synthesis

Pancreas
• Insulin secretion

NIGHT

Muscle
• Oxidative metabolism

Fat
• Lipid catabolism
• Leptin secretion

Liver
• Gluconeogenesis
• Glycogenolysis
• Mitochondrial biogenesis

Pancreas
• Glucagon secretion

References:

Reddy, S. (2022, March 23). Why Permanent Daylight-Saving Time Is Bad for Your Health, Sleep Scientists Say. WSJ. https://www.wsj.com/articles/why-permanent-daylight-saving-time-is-bad-for-your-health-sleep-scientists-say-11648002326?mod=Searchresults_pos2&page=1

https://www.google.com/url?sa=i&url=https%3A%2F%2Fcommons.wikimedia.org%2Fwiki%2FFile%3AThe_master_circadian_clock_in_the_human_brain.jpg&psig=AOvVaw3TSBGxCBA6-sRuo0ptw5Nv&ust=1649364016576000&source=images&cd=vfe&ved=0CAoQjRxqFwoTCMio_falgPcCFQAAAAAdAAAAABAr

Leone, M., Campbell, J., & Moltzan, J. (2022, July 26). Journey Around the Sun-2nd Edition (Health and Wellness Study Guides Using Eastern Practices from Martial Arts, Yoga and Qigong). CAD Graphics.

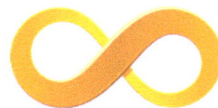

Social media has become an integral part of modern life, offering a platform for self-expression, networking, and information sharing. However, when individuals, especially those with professional careers, use social media to constantly post their political and social views, it can lead to unintended consequences. This behavior, particularly when it involves posting dozens of times a day with little engagement, can be polarizing and may negatively impact both personal and professional relationships. Beyond the social and professional risks, this kind of behavior can also have significant psychological and physiological effects, including stress, cortisol imbalances, and even obsessive-compulsive tendencies.

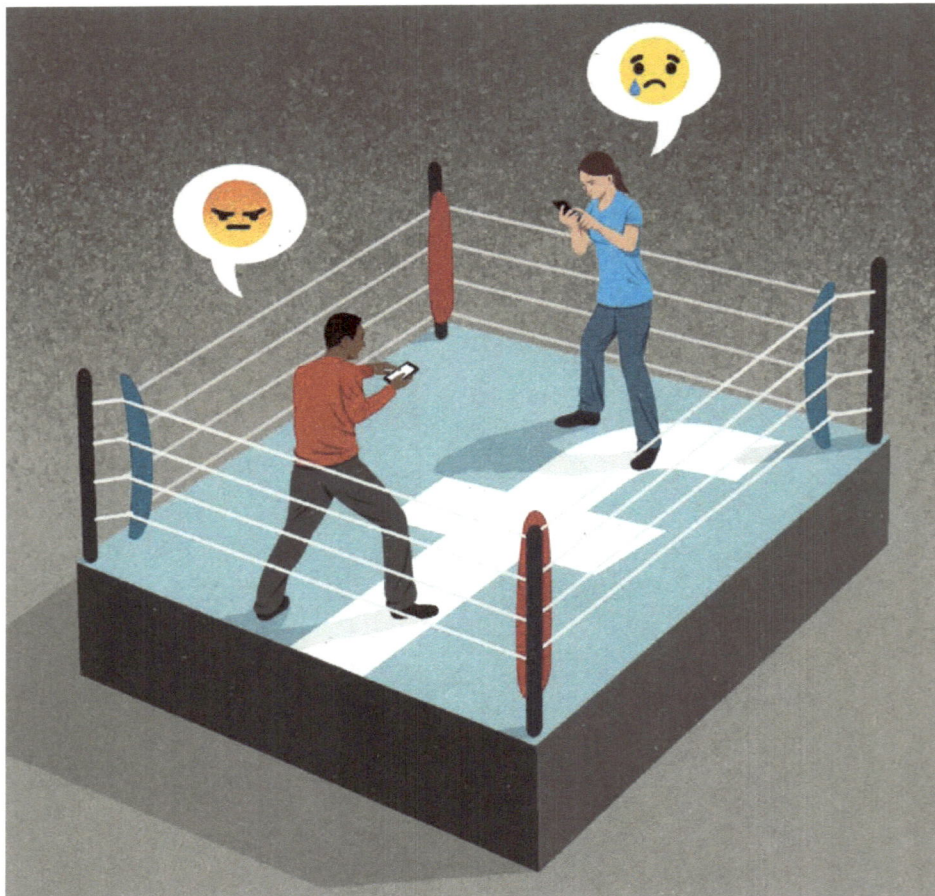

https://www.wsj.com/articles/why-social-media-is-so-good-at-polarizing-us-11603105204

Professional Risks

One of the most immediate detriments of excessive posting of polarizing views is the potential harm to one's professional reputation. For individuals with established careers, social media often extends their professional identity. When their online presence is dominated by divisive political or social commentary, it can overshadow their expertise and accomplishments. Colleagues, clients, or professional networks with differing views may feel alienated, leading to strained relationships or missed opportunities. In extreme cases, this behavior can even result in job loss or damage to one's career trajectory, as employers increasingly scrutinize employees' online activity.

Engagement and Feedback

Another notable issue is the lack of engagement these posts often receive. When individuals post frequently and assertively, framing their views as absolute truths, it can discourage others from responding. People may find the content unrelatable, exhausting, or confrontational, leading to a lack of meaningful dialogue. Over time, this can create an echo chamber where the individual only hears their own voice, further entrenching their beliefs and isolating them from diverse perspectives. This lack of engagement can also be a sign that their approach is counterproductive, as it fails to foster the kind of constructive conversations that could lead to mutual understanding.

Do US Adults Think That Social Media Has More of a Positive or Negative Effect on Their Own Mental Health?

% of respondents, by generation, Feb 2023

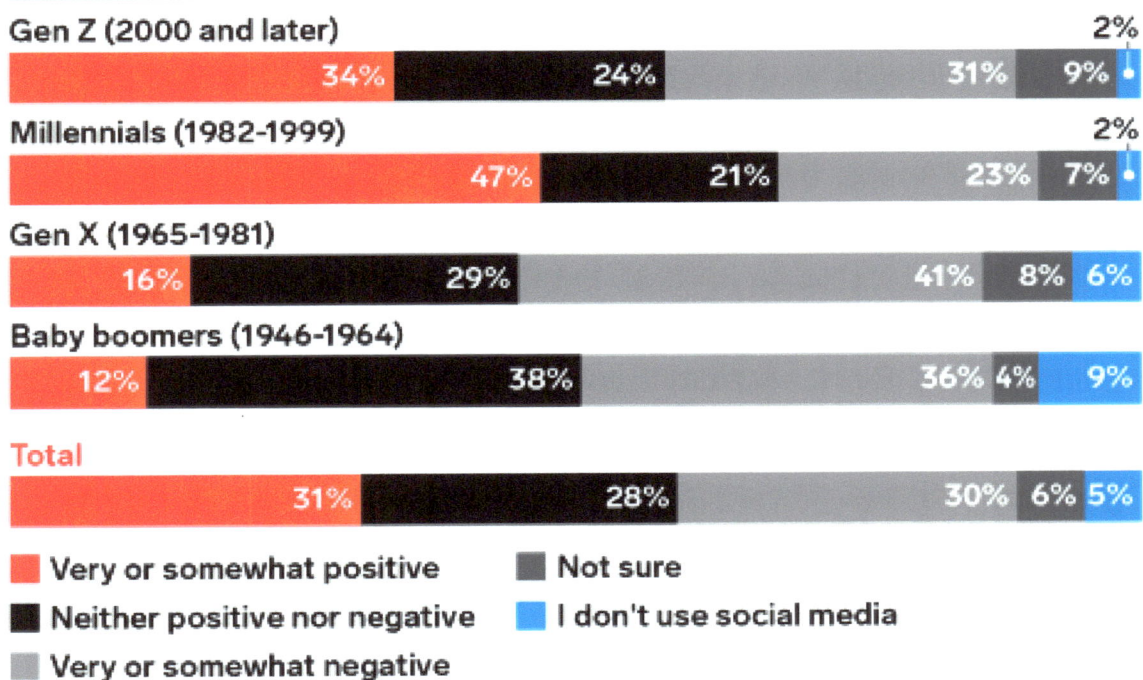

Gen Z (2000 and later)

| 34% | 24% | 31% | 9% | 2% |

Millennials (1982-1999)

| 47% | 21% | 23% | 7% | 2% |

Gen X (1965-1981)

| 16% | 29% | 41% | 8% | 6% |

Baby boomers (1946-1964)

| 12% | 38% | 36% | 4% | 9% |

Total

| 31% | 28% | 30% | 6% | 5% |

- ■ Very or somewhat positive
- ■ Neither positive nor negative
- ■ Very or somewhat negative
- ■ Not sure
- ■ I don't use social media

Source: YouGov as cited in company blog, March 11, 2023

280945　　　InsiderIntelligence.com

https://www.emarketer.com/content/social-media-boost-mental-health-millennials

118

A Shift in How We Engage with Perspectives

In the past, before the advent of social media, people often engaged in face-to-face conversations where curiosity about others' perspectives was more common. There was a natural inclination to ask questions, listen, and seek to understand differing viewpoints. Social media, however, has fundamentally altered this dynamic. Today, we are freely able and often inundated with the thoughts and opinions of others, sometimes to the point of oversaturation. While this transparency can foster connection, it can also lead to fatigue, especially when those opinions are expressed aggressively or excessively. The mystery and curiosity that once fueled meaningful dialogue are often replaced by a sense of overexposure, where the sheer volume of content can make it difficult to engage thoughtfully.

Psychological and Emotional Impact

The psychological and emotional toll of this behavior cannot be overlooked. Constantly posting polarizing content may stem from a deep-seated need for validation or a desire to influence others. However, when these posts go unnoticed or unacknowledged, it can lead to feelings of frustration, inadequacy, or even anger. Over time, this cycle can contribute to heightened stress levels and emotional exhaustion. Moreover, the act of repeatedly sharing strong opinions can become compulsive, resembling obsessive-compulsive tendencies. The individual may feel an uncontrollable urge to post, even when it no longer serves a constructive purpose. If someone has the time, effort, and energy to blame others for all of the world's ills, they also have the time to reflect and focus on becoming a better version of themselves. Rather than dwelling on external problems, shifting some of that energy toward self-improvement could yield far more positive and constructive outcomes.

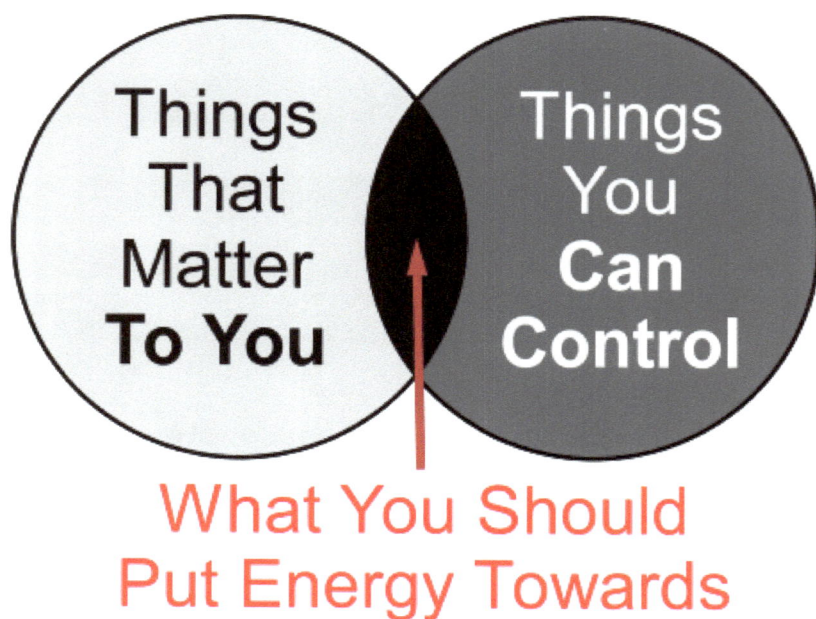

Things That Matter To You / Things You Can Control

What You Should Put Energy Towards

Respecting Passion Without Sharing It

It's worth noting that while someone's efforts to advocate for a cause may appear noble or well-intentioned, not everyone will share their passion or agree with their methods. Social media often amplifies the visibility of these efforts, making it seem as though everyone should be equally invested. However, it's important to recognize that people have different priorities, values, and capacities for engagement. What one person sees as a critical issue worthy of relentless advocacy, another may view as less pressing or outside their sphere of interest. This disconnect doesn't diminish the value of the cause itself, but it highlights the importance of respecting boundaries and understanding that not everyone will share the same level of enthusiasm or commitment.

Physiological Effects: Stress, Cortisol, and Chemical Imbalances

The psychological stress associated with excessive social media use can also manifest physiologically. Chronic stress triggers the release of cortisol, a hormone that, in excess, can disrupt the body's natural balance. Elevated cortisol levels have been linked to a range of health issues, including anxiety, depression, sleep disturbances, and weakened immune function. For individuals who are constantly engaged in online debates or who feel compelled to post frequently, this stress response can become a persistent state, leading to long-term health consequences.

CHEAP DOPAMINE   REAL DOPAMINE

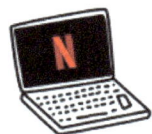 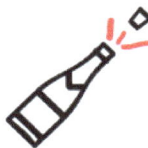 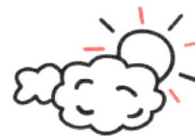 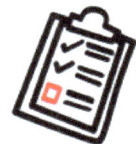

SERIES / TV   ALCOHOL   JUNK FOOD   NEW   SUN &   WORK ON
                                            EXPERIENCES   OUTDOORS   YOUR GOALS

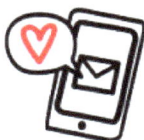 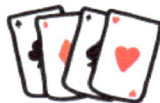 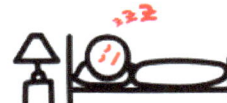 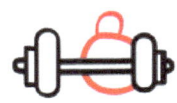

DRUGS   SOCIAL MEDIA   GAMBLING   REST   GOOD SLEEP   EXERCISE

Additionally, the dopamine-driven nature of social media can exacerbate these issues. The anticipation of likes, shares, or comments triggers dopamine release, reinforcing a habit loop. Over time, this can contribute to compulsive posting, as individuals seek continued validation through online interactions. This chemical imbalance can make it difficult for individuals to step away from social media, even when they recognize its negative impact on their lives.

Constructive Approaches for Change

For individuals who find themselves caught in this cycle, there are steps they can take to create a healthier and more balanced online presence. First, they might consider diversifying their content to include professional achievements, personal interests, or neutral topics that encourage broader engagement. Framing opinions in a way that invites dialogue—such as asking, "What are your thoughts on this?"—can also foster more respectful and productive conversations. Additionally, limiting the frequency of posts and focusing on quality over quantity can help reduce the compulsive urge to share and create a more thoughtful online presence.

For Observers: Setting Boundaries and Offering Support

For those who are on the receiving end of this behavior, it's important to set boundaries. If the constant stream of polarizing posts becomes overwhelming, muting or unfollowing the individual on social media can help maintain mental well-being while preserving professional relationships. It's also helpful to remember that their behavior is likely a reflection of their own experiences and beliefs, not a personal attack. In some cases, offering constructive feedback—if the relationship allows—can encourage them to reflect on their approach and its impact on others.

Conclusion

While social media offers a powerful platform for self-expression, its misuse can have far-reaching consequences. For individuals who post their political and social views excessively, the risks include professional alienation, strained relationships, and psychological and physiological harm. By adopting a more balanced and thoughtful approach to social media, individuals can mitigate these detriments and create a more positive and productive online presence. For observers, setting boundaries and offering support can help navigate these challenging dynamics. Ultimately, social media is a tool, and its impact depends on how it is used. By using social media intentionally and fostering meaningful discussions rather than divisive debates, we can create a digital space that informs rather than isolates.

References:

Mims, C., & Holcroft, J. (2020, October 19). Why social media is so good at polarizing us. *WSJ*. https://www.wsj.com/articles/why-social-media-is-so-good-at-polarizing-us-11603105204

Professional Risks of Social Media Use

Brown, V. R., & Vaughn, E. D. (2011). *The writing on the (Facebook) wall: The use of social networking sites in hiring decisions.* Journal of Business and Psychology, 26(2), 219-225.

- This study explores how employers evaluate candidates' social media presence and the potential impact of polarizing content.

Echo Chambers and Engagement Issues

Pariser, E. (2011). *The Filter Bubble: What the Internet Is Hiding from You.* Penguin Press.
- Discusses how social media algorithms reinforce pre-existing beliefs and limit exposure to diverse perspectives.

Psychological and Emotional Effects of Social Media Overuse

Twenge, J. M., Joiner, T. E., Rogers, M. L., & Martin, G. N. (2017). Increases in depressive Symptoms, Suicide-Related Outcomes, and suicide rates among U.S. adolescents after 2010 and links to increased new media screen time. *Clinical Psychological Science*, 6(1), 3–17. https://doi.org/10.1177/2167702617723376

- Examines how excessive screen time and social media use contribute to stress, anxiety, and depression.

Physiological Impact: Stress, Cortisol, and Dopamine

Sapolsky, R. M. (2004). *Why Zebras Don't Get Ulcers.* Holt Paperbacks.
- Explains how chronic stress and elevated cortisol levels affect mental and physical health.

Montag, C., & Reuter, M. (2017). *Internet Addiction: Neuroscientific Approaches and Therapeutical Implications Including Smartphone Addiction.* Springer.
- Discusses dopamine-driven social media addiction and its effect on brain function.

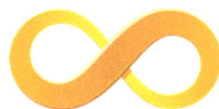

In Traditional Chinese Medicine (TCM), the human body is seen not merely as a collection of parts but as an interconnected system of energy, spirit, emotion, and function. One of the most profound concepts in TCM is that each major organ system is linked to a particular emotion. Among these, the **Heart** is associated with the emotion of **Joy,** a connection that is both beautiful and cautionary.

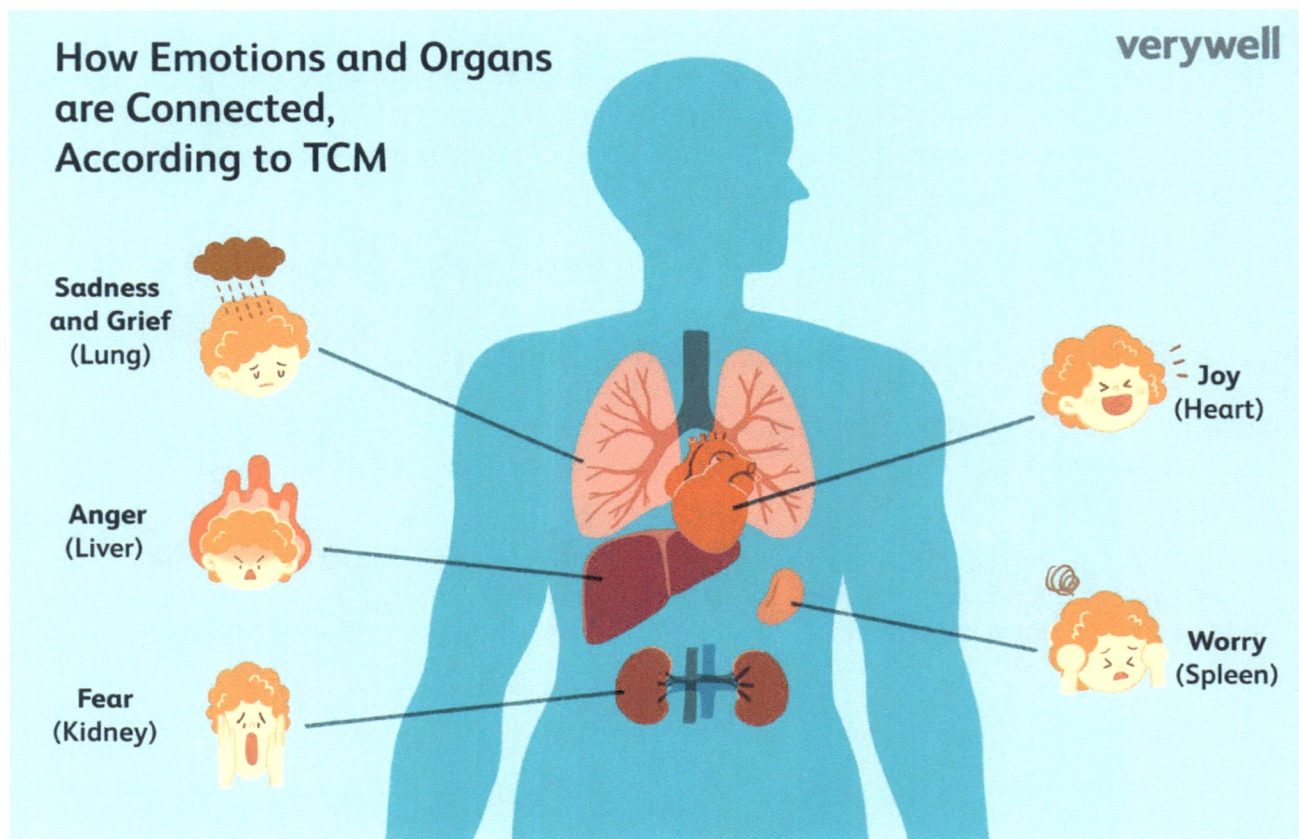

(Vanbuskirk, 2024)

The Heart: Emperor of the Organ Systems

According to classical TCM, the Heart is not just a mechanical pump. It is the "Emperor" of the body's organ systems. It governs the blood and blood vessels, controls the tongue, and most significantly, houses the *Shen* the mind or spirit.

Heart Correspondences:
- **Element**: Fire

- **Season**: Summer

- **Color**: Red

- **Flavor**: Bitter

- **Tissue**: Blood vessels

- **Sense Organ**: Tongue

- **Emotion**: Joy

- **Spirit**: Shen (Mind/Spirit)

When the Heart is balanced, we experience mental clarity, restful sleep, appropriate excitement, and the capacity for deep connection with others.

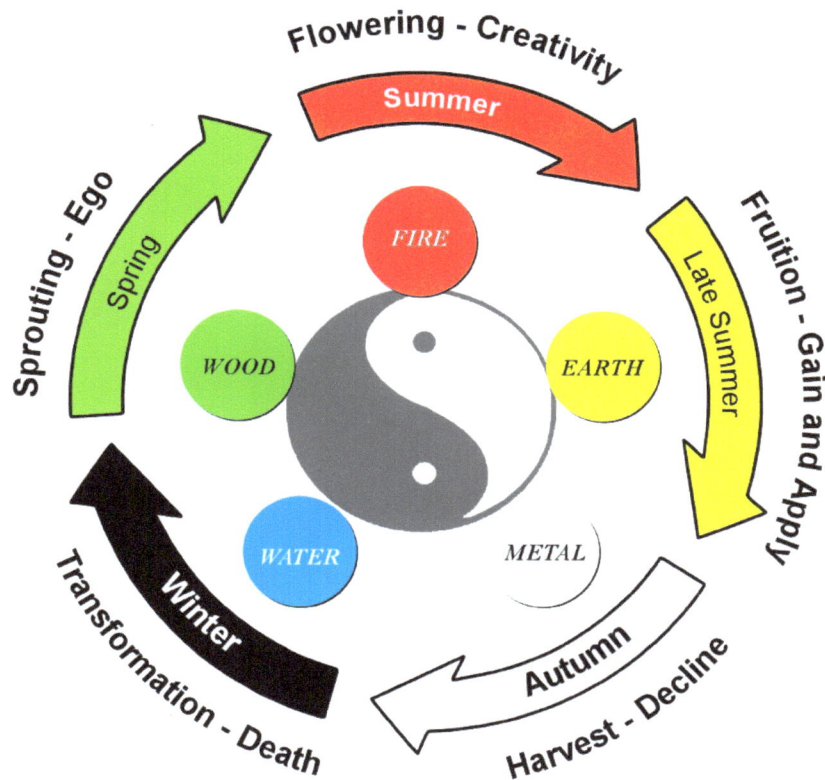

Joy: The Nourishing Emotion

In appropriate doses, joy is a deeply nourishing force. Joy:
- Soothes the nervous system and eases emotional tension

- Promotes circulatory warmth and a sense of connection

- Lifts the Shen, resulting in laughter, optimism, and creativity

- It is vital to a healthy spiritual life

Joy reflects the expansive nature of the Fire element. Like the sun in summer, it radiates outward, illuminating relationships and animating the spirit.

When Joy Becomes Excessive

Paradoxically, the very emotion that nourishes the Heart can also harm it when excessive or poorly regulated. In TCM, "excess joy" includes:
- Overexcitement, mania, or hysteria
- Hyperactivity, constant stimulation
- Overindulgence in pleasure or celebration

Physiological Consequences of Excess Joy:
- **Scattering of the Shen**: The mind becomes ungrounded or erratic.
- **Heart Qi disruption**: Can result in palpitations, insomnia, anxiety.
- **Mental-emotional disturbances**: Talkativeness, inappropriate laughter, dream-disturbed sleep.

In modern terms, this may resemble bipolar mania, panic disorder, or emotional exhaustion. Prolonged joy without rest can overheat the system, especially in individuals already constitutionally "hot" or deficient in Yin.

The Importance of Emotional Balance in TCM
TCM recognizes no emotion as inherently negative. Emotions are considered physiological energies that must move freely, but in balance.

Emotion	Organ System	In Balance	In Excess
Joy	Heart	Warmth, clarity, connection	Scattered mind, insomnia, palpitations
Anger	Liver	Motivation, assertiveness	Irritability, tension, high blood pressure
Worry	Spleen	Compassion, thoughtfulness	Obsession, overthinking, fatigue
Grief	Lung	Reverence, release	Depression, breathlessness
Fear	Kidney	Caution, intuition	Panic, low back pain, adrenal fatigue

All five emotions (and their corresponding organ systems) influence one another. For example, chronic overstimulation (excess joy) may weaken the Heart and eventually impact on the Kidneys (fear) or the Spleen (overthinking), leading to broader emotional and physical disharmony.

Recognizing Heart-Shen Imbalance

Signs that joy has turned from nourishing to disruptive may include:
- Insomnia or difficulty falling asleep

- Restlessness or excessive chatter

- Palpitations or fluttering heartbeat

- Red tip of the tongue (Heart Fire sign)

- Vivid or disturbing dreams

- Uncontrollable laughter or emotional outbursts

Practitioners aim to calm the Shen, clear Heart Fire, and nourish Heart Yin with techniques such as:
- Acupuncture (e.g., Heart 7, Pericardium 6)

- Herbal formulas (e.g., Tian Wang Bu Xin Dan)

- Meditation and breathwork

- Avoidance of overstimulation, especially in summer

A Holistic Reflection

In the West, joy is often pursued as a goal in itself. But TCM offers a subtle reminder: true wellness lies not in constant happiness but in dynamic balance. Joy, like fire, is beautiful but unchecked, it can burn.

Instead of constant excitement, TCM encourages us to cultivate:
- Contentment

- Presence

- Inner peace

By anchoring our joy in stillness, we allow the Shen to rest peacefully in the Heart, just as the sun sets each day to allow the body to restore.

References:

Kaptchuk, T. J. (2000). *The Web That Has No Weaver: Understanding Chinese Medicine*. McGraw-Hill.

Vanbuskirk, S. (2024, October 25). How emotions and organs are connected in traditional Chinese medicine. Verywell Mind. https://www.verywellmind.com/emotions-in-traditional-chinese-medicine-88196

SECTION VI: BREATHWORK & CONSCIOUSNESS

Slow Breathing, why is This Beneficial?

Internal practices like *tai chi, qigong*, and *yoga* that encourage slow, deep breathing can *enhance* rather than hinder oxygen delivery and energy during physically demanding postures. Let me unpack how this works from a Western physiological perspective, while also nodding to the energetic logic behind these practices.

Physiological Mechanisms at Play

1. Low Breathing Rate ≠ Low Oxygen Intake
- When breathing frequency is reduced *intentionally*, it's usually paired with deeper, more diaphragmatic breaths (also called "belly breathing").

- This increases tidal volume (the amount of air per breath), so although you're breathing fewer times per minute, you may be getting the same or even more oxygen overall.

- Slower breathing also enhances alveolar gas exchange because air stays in the lungs longer, allowing more thorough oxygen and CO_2 exchange.

Normal respiration rate: ~12 to 15 breaths/min (18 or more BPM when stressed)
In skilled practice: ~4–6 breaths/min (or less), with full exhalation and longer pause phases

2. Parasympathetic Activation and Efficiency
- Slow, conscious breathing activates the parasympathetic nervous system (rest and digest), which:
  - Slows heart rate
  - Lowers blood pressure
  - Enhances vasodilation (better blood flow to extremities)

- This reduces physiological tension, allowing the muscles to function more efficiently with less oxygen demand per unit of work.

3. Increased CO_2 Tolerance and Oxygen Utilization
- Practices that involve breath retention or very slow breathing increase carbon dioxide (CO_2) tolerance.

- Contrary to popular belief, CO_2 is the key signal for oxygen release via the Bohr effect:
  - Higher CO_2 levels shift hemoglobin to release more O_2 into tissues.

- So, by tolerating higher CO_2, you actually increase oxygen delivery where it's needed, especially in muscles under tension.

4. Improved Circulatory and Lymphatic Flow

- Many postures in tai chi, yoga, and qigong involve dynamic tension, twisting, and limb positioning that:
    - Gently compress and release blood vessels (like a pump)
    - Aid in venous return (blood going back to the heart)
    - Enhance lymphatic drainage, helping with detox and immune function
- Combined with deep breathing (which changes intra-thoracic pressure), these techniques mimic a second circulatory pump, where the breath and posture work together.

5. Enhanced Proprioception and Motor Control

- By slowing breath and motion, practitioners become more aware of subtle muscle activation and joint positioning.
- The cerebellum and somatosensory cortex are engaged more deeply, improving neuromuscular efficiency, so less "effort" is needed for the same or better results.
- Muscles co-contract (*yin-yang* balance) with greater harmony, reducing unnecessary energy output.

Energetic and Traditional Viewpoint

From Traditional Chinese Medicine (TCM) or yogic perspectives:
- Breath (*qi/prana*) is not just oxygen; it's vital energy that nourishes tissues.
- Slower breathing "builds" qi rather than expending it.
- Holding postures while breathing deeply and slowly opens energy meridians, improves energy flow, and harmonizes internal organs.
- In yoga, this aligns with *pranayama* and *bandhas* (locks), which store and redirect prana rather than dissipating it.

Slow Breathing Increases Wellness During Internal Practices of Tai Chi, Qigong, Yoga

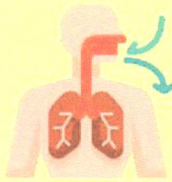

Slower Breathing
Respiration rate ▼   tidal volume ▲

offers better gas exchange & oxygen delivery

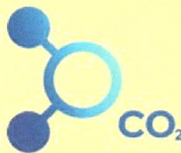

CO_2 Tolerance
CO_2 ▲ (Bohr effect)

offers better O_2 release to muscles

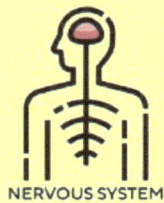

Parasympathetic Activation
Heart Rate ▼ Blood Pressure ▼ vasodilation ▲

offers more efficient muscle use

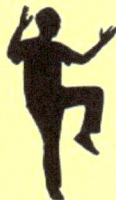

Postural Effects
Muscle tension + breathing

offers better venous return + lymph drainage

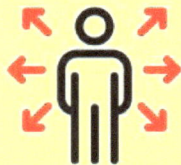

Neuromuscular Control
Proprioception ▲

offers less wasted effort

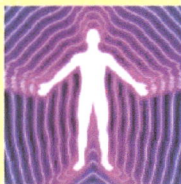

Energetic Flow
Qi/Prana builds through slow breath & posture
offering less depletion

Summary: Why It Works

Challenge	Physiological Adaptation
Low breath rate under tension	Increased tidal volume, better gas exchange
Increased CO_2	Enhanced oxygen delivery via Bohr effect
Muscle demand	Greater circulatory efficiency, less waste buildup
Nervous system stress	Parasympathetic dominance reduces overexertion
Static/dynamic postures	Lymphatic drainage, better venous return
Breath–movement harmony	Improved motor control, proprioception, energetic alignment

References:

Brown, R. P., & Gerbarg, P. L. (2005). Sudarshan Kriya Yogic Breathing in the Treatment of Stress, Anxiety, and Depression: Part II—Clinical Applications and Guidelines. *The Journal of Alternative and Complementary Medicine*, *11*(4), 711–717. https://doi.org/10.1089/acm.2005.11.711

Jerath, R., Edry, J. W., Barnes, V. A., & Jerath, V. (2006). Physiology of long pranayamic breathing: Neural respiratory elements may provide a mechanism that explains how slow deep breathing shifts the autonomic nervous system. *Medical Hypotheses*, *67*(3), 566–571. https://doi.org/10.1016/j.mehy.2006.02.042

Bernardi, L., Gabutti, A., Porta, C., & Spicuzza, L. (2001).

Slow breathing reduces chemoreflex response to hypoxia and hypercapnia, and increases baroreflex sensitivity. *Journal of Hypertension, 19*(12), 2221–2229. https://doi.org/10.1097/00004872-200112000-00016

Slow breathing reduces chemoreflex response to hypoxia and. . . : Journal of Hypertension. (n.d.). LWW. https://journals.lww.com/jhypertension/abstract/2001/12000/slow_breathing_reduces_chemoreflex_response_to.16.aspx

Streeter, C., Gerbarg, P., Saper, R., Ciraulo, D., & Brown, R. (2012). Effects of yoga on the autonomic nervous system, gamma-aminobutyric-acid, and allostasis in epilepsy, depression, and post-traumatic stress disorder. *Medical Hypotheses*, *78*(5), 571–579. https://doi.org/10.1016/j.mehy.2012.01.021

Lehrer, P. M., & Gevirtz, R. (2014). Heart rate variability biofeedback: how and why does it work? *Frontiers in Psychology*, *5*. https://doi.org/10.3389/fpsyg.2014.00756

The Importance of Nose Breathing

There is evidence that breathing through the nose creates air oscillations which can increase nitric oxide (NO) through the rise in exchange of air between the nasal cavity and the paranasal sinuses. The paranasal sinuses can then produce larger amounts of nitric oxide which increases oxygen uptake. Nitric oxide is a powerful and potent vasodilator. Pulmonary Vascular Resistance (PVR) was shown in research studies to be reduced during nasal breathing when compared to mouth breathing. Additionally, nitric oxide aids in nonspecific host defense against infections stemming from bacteria, viruses, fungi, and parasites (Trivedi & Saboo, 2021).

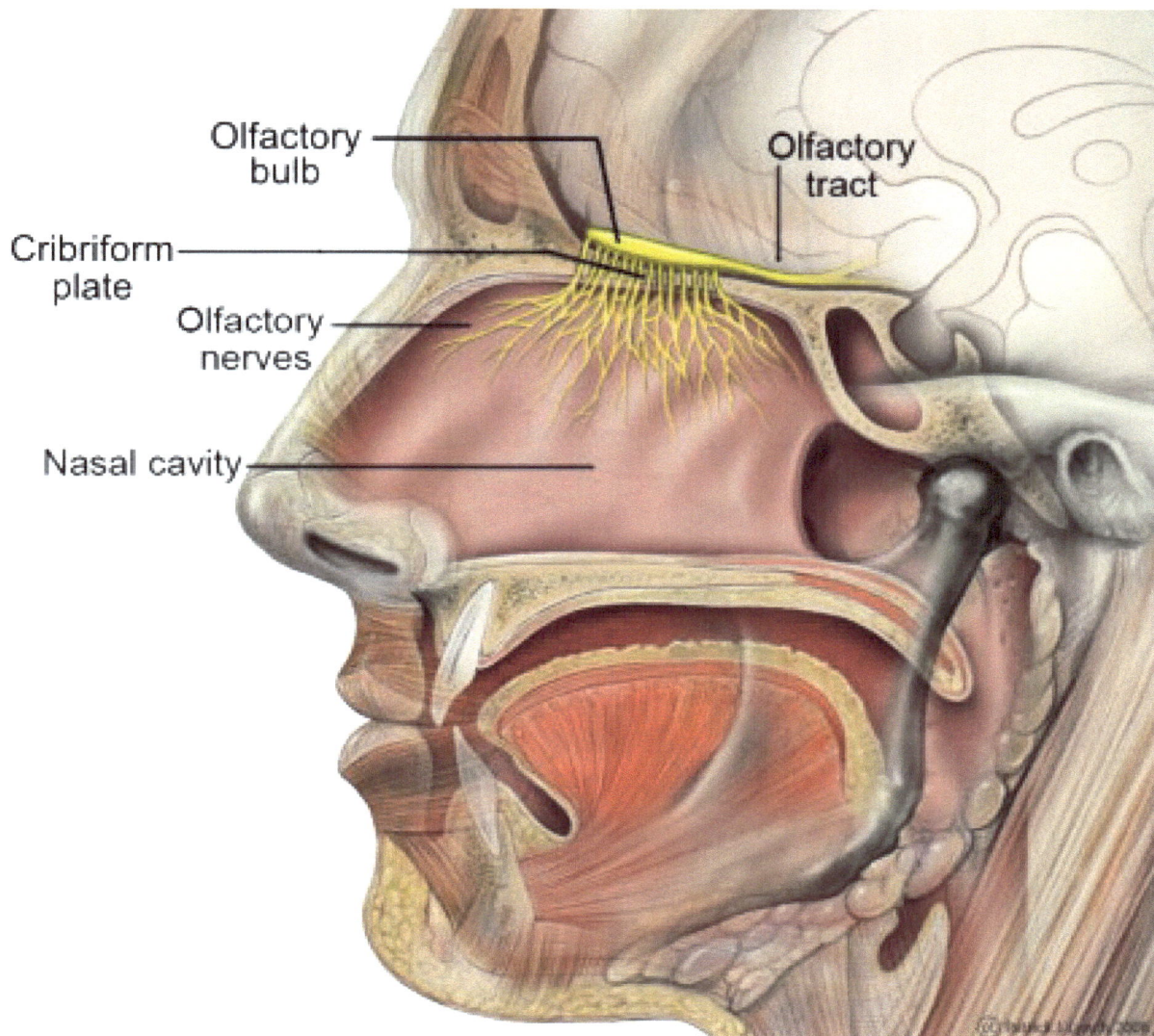

In 1988, the Nobel Prize in Physiology was awarded to Robert F. Furchgott of the State University of New York Health Science Center in Brooklyn, Ferid Murad of the University of Texas Medical School in Houston, and Louis J. Ignarro of the University of California School of Medicine in Los Angeles. The award was for their discoveries regarding nitric oxide as a signaling molecule in the cardiovascular system.

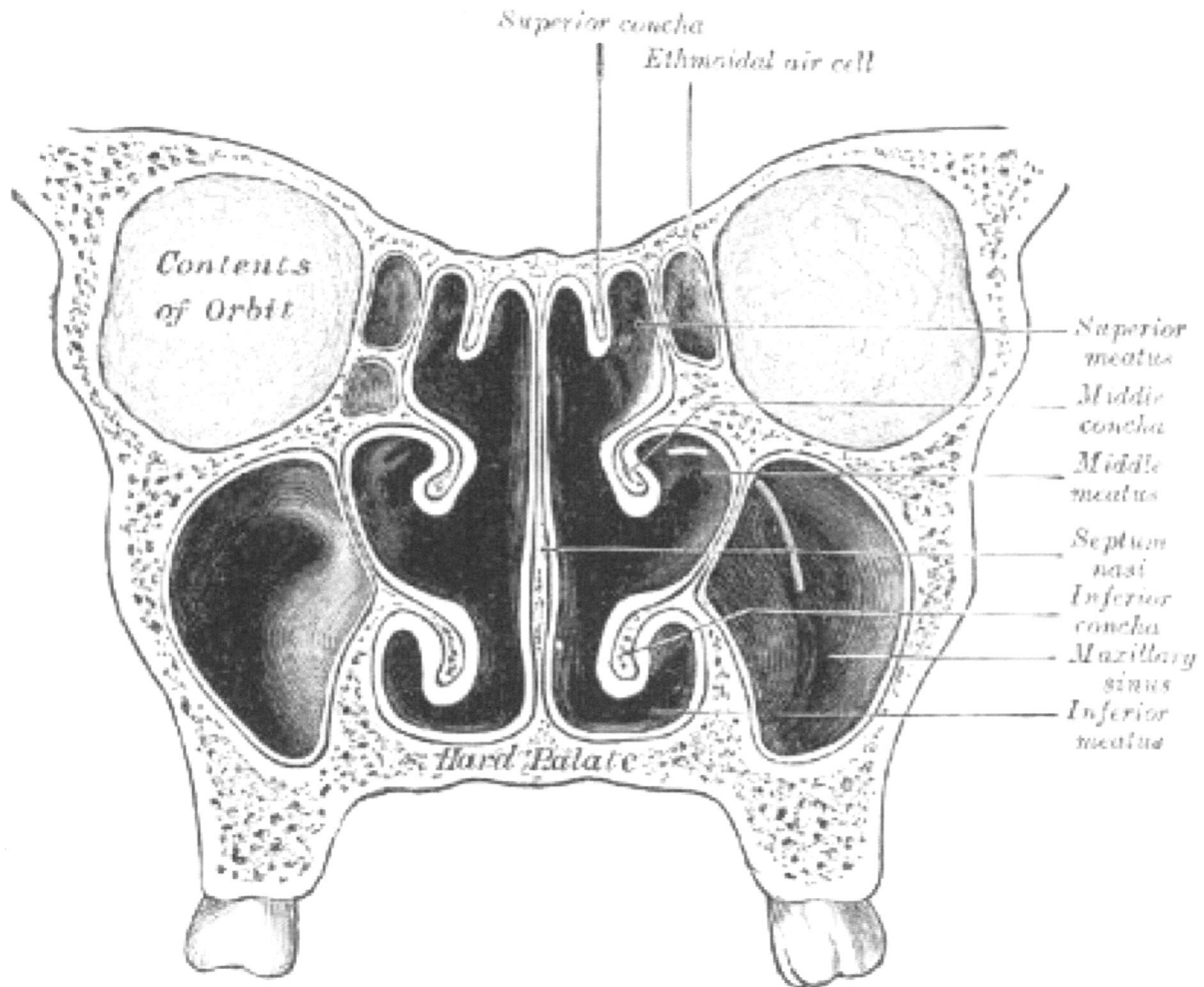

Furchgott had previously discovered that endothelial cells that line the interior blood vessels, produce this signaling molecule of nitric oxide (NO). NO makes nearby muscles relax and consequently help to regulate blood pressure. More recently, scientists have discovered that the enzymes with which cells make the short-lived gas play a role in activities such as immunity, memory formation, and tumor suppression. Some brain cells also send messages using NO. Immune cells release bursts of nitric oxide to kill infectious organisms and cancer cells. Doctors are also researching the effects of nitric oxide with premature infants to stimulate blood flow to their underdeveloped lungs (Travis, 1998).

Nitric Oxide
(NO)

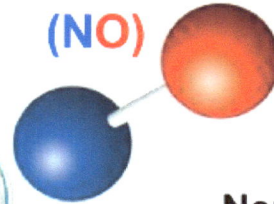

Vision
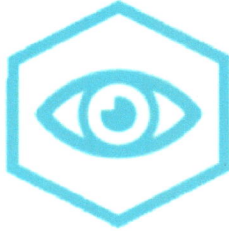
- neurotransmitter within retina
- regulation of retinal blood flow
- visual transduction
- effector in photoreceptors
- muscle tone in retinal and choroidal circulation

Cardiovascular System
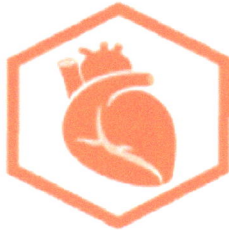
- opening of blood vessels
- blood cell health
- heart strength
- nutrient exchange

Respiratory System
- Bronchial dilation
- Pulmonary vascular reactivity
- Alveolar-capillary membrane permeability

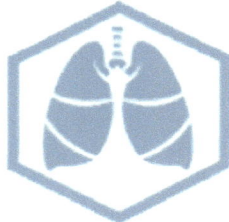

Neurological System
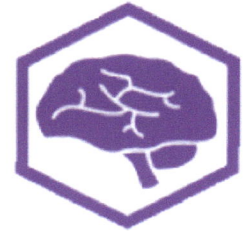
- Learning
- Memory
- Neural protection
- Neuronal toxicity
- Neurotransmission
- Neuronal development
- Nociception
- enhances "rest stste"
- pain management
- blood pressure regulation

Urogenital System
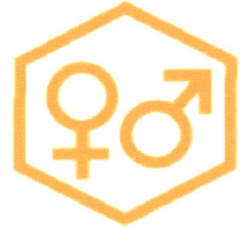
- reninsecretion
- penile erection
- fertilization
- spermatogenisis, oogenesis, ovulation

Excretory System
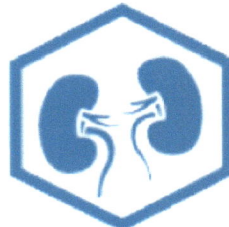
- Glomerular filtration
- Renal vasodilation
- Renal endothelial function

Endocrine System
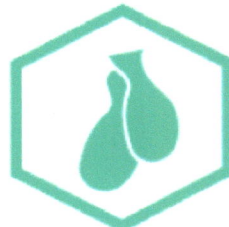
- posterior pituitary hormones
- gonadotropin hypothalamic releasing factor

Immune System
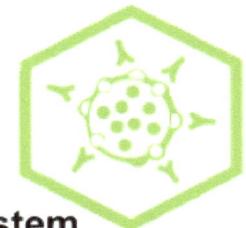
- improved Innate immunity
- inflammation regulation
- cytotoxic chemical
- cellular injury protection
- superoxide radical quenching

Gastrointestinal Tract
- enhanced metabolism
- increases nutrient absorption

Cell Proliferation
- reduced cell death
- new blood vessel formation

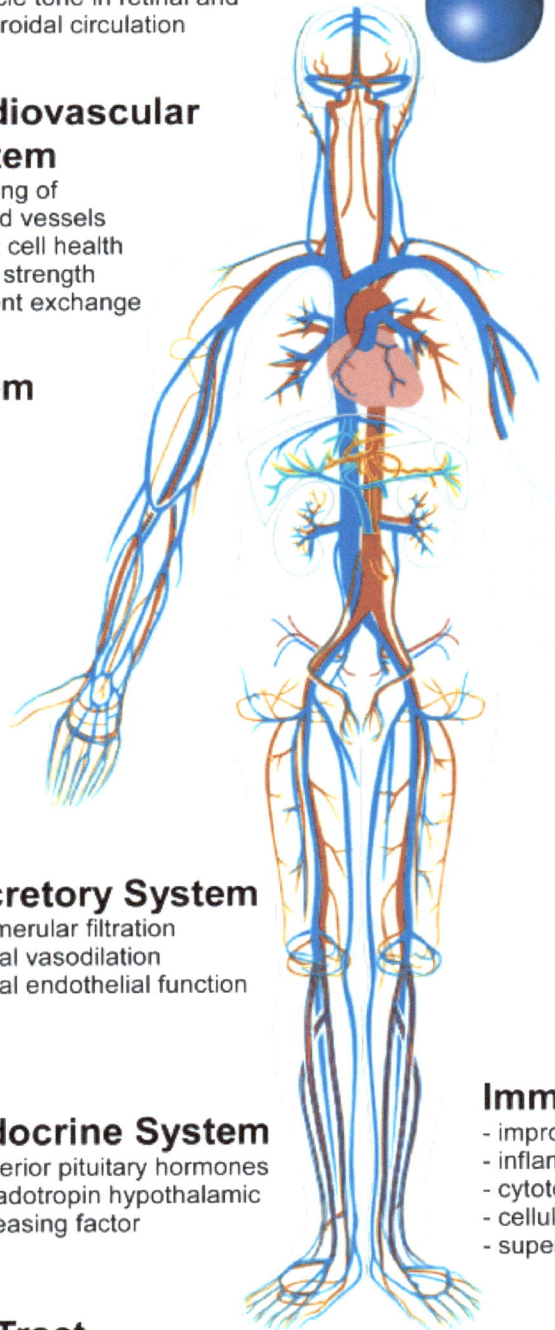

(c) Copyright 2022 - CAD Graphics, Inc

www.MindandBodyExercises.com

134

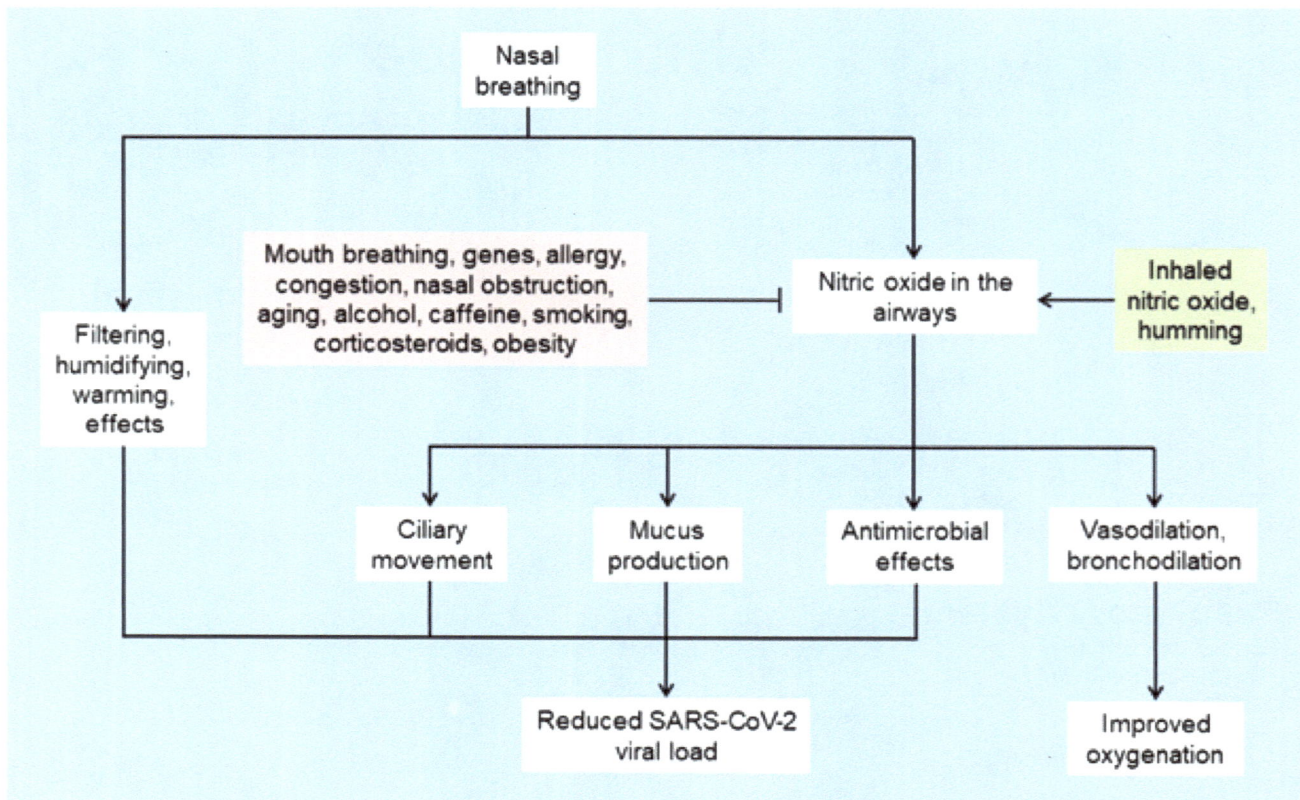

https://learntosleepwell.com/scientific-research/could-nasal-nitric-oxide-help-to-mitigate-the-severity-of-covid-19/

Yoga (qigong), tai chi, meditation, martial arts and other methods often put a major emphasis on regulated breathing through the nose.

References:

Trivedi, G. Y., & Saboo, B. (2021). Bhramari Pranayama – A simple lifestyle intervention to reduce heart rate, enhance the lung function and immunity. Journal of Ayurveda and Integrative Medicine, 12(3), 562–564. https://doi-org.northernvermont.idm.oclc.org/10.1016/j.jaim.2021.07.004

Travis, J. (1998, October 17). Medical Nobel prize says yes to NO. (nitric oxide research honored)(Brief Article). Science News, v154(n16), p246.

YOU'VE BEEN BREATHING ALL WRONG: Hey mouth-breathers! Use your nose to boost immunity–and mood.(SCIENCE). (2020, July 1). Maclean's, 133(6), 76.

SETTERGREN, ANGDIN, ASTUDILLO, GELINDER, LISKA, LUNDBERG, WEITZBERG, & Settergren, G. (1998). Decreased pulmonary vascular resistance during nasal breathing: modulation by endogenous nitric oxide from the paranasal sinuses. Acta Physiologica Scandinavica, 163(3), 235–239.

Struben, V. M. D., Wieringa, M. H., Mantingh, C. J., Bruinsma, S. M., de Jongste, J. C., & Feenstra, L. (2005). Silent and humming nasal NO measurements in adults aged 18–70 years. European Journal of Clinical Investigation, 35(10), 653–657. https://doi-org.northernvermont.idm.oclc.org/10.1111/j.1365-2362.2005.01559.x

Ethmoid Bone – Location – Structure – Relationships. (2020, December 5). TeachMeAnatomy. https://teachmeanatomy.info/head/osteology/ethmoid-bone/

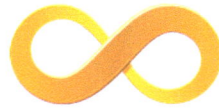

Nose Breathing vs. Mouth Breathing

Among many healthcare professionals, fitness enthusiasts, martial artists, musical instrument performers, and others understand that breathing through the nose, or nasal breathing is generally considered better than breathing solely through the mouth for several reasons:

1. Improved Air Filtration
Moist nasal passages help to filter pollen, dust, pathogens, and other allergens through tiny hairs called cilia and mucus which protect the lungs from harmful particles.

2. Increased Oxygen Absorption
Nasal breathing can slow down the rate of airflow, allowing more time for oxygen exchange in the lungs. This consequently leads to better oxygen delivery to tissues.

3. Better Air Humidification and Temperature Regulation
The nasal passages warm and humidify incoming air, helping to reduce irritation to the respiratory tract and improving overall comfort, particularly in dry or cold climates.

4. Nitric Oxide Production
Nitric oxide (NO) is a vital key messenger molecule produced in the endothelium found inside our blood vessels. As a vasodilator NO modulates vascular tone, which enhances healthy blood flow and circulation, and is a key to overall physiological organ function. NO affects blood pressure, vitality, and nutrient absorption which impacts many aspects of health. As blood vessels dilate, blood flow increases to improve exercise performance and improve brain function. The nasal sinuses provide a very large reservoir of nitric oxide (NO). Nasal breathing stimulates nitric oxide production, improving oxygen levels throughout the body. Yoga (qigong), tai chi, meditation, martial arts and other methods often put a major emphasis on regulated breathing through the nose.

5. Supports Proper Diaphragmatic Breathing
Nasal breathing encourages deeper, more controlled breathing, activating the respiratory diaphragm and reducing shallow, chest-dominated breaths often associated with stress.

6. Better Sleep Quality
Nasal breathing reduces snoring and thus reduces the risk of sleep apnea, promoting more restful and restorative sleep.

7. Improved Oral Health

Keeping the mouth closed during breathing is thought to prevent dry mouth, reducing the risk of cavities, gum disease, and bad breath.

8. Enhancement of Athletic Performance
Nasal breathing increases endurance and efficient energy use, by improving oxygen uptake and reducing the buildup of carbon dioxide within the bloodstream.

9. Balanced CO_2 and Oxygen Levels
Breathing through the nose helps maintain an optimal balance of carbon dioxide and oxygen in the blood, supporting cellular metabolism and calming the nervous system.

10. Supports Facial Development (in Children)
In children, nasal breathing promotes proper tongue posture and jaw development, reducing the risk of orthodontic issues and improving facial structure.

11. Promotes Postural Alignment
Nasal breathing supports proper tongue posture, which can improve overall posture and reduce strain on the neck and back.

12. Reduced Stress and Anxiety
Nasal breathing activates the parasympathetic nervous system, which helps reduce heart rate and stress levels, promoting a calm and focused state of mind.

13. Boosts Cognitive Function
Consistent oxygen distribution to the brain enhances focus, memory, and decision-making capabilities.

14. Voice Quality and Speech Clarity
Maintaining nasal breathing increases vocal cord health and improves voice resonance and clarity.

There may be situations where breathing through the mouth is necessary or preferable, such as during intense physical exertion or when experiencing nasal congestion. However, nasal breathing is considered the more natural and physiologically advantageous way to breathe. If someone experiences chronic nasal congestion or other issues that impede nasal breathing, it's advisable to consult with a healthcare professional.

Box Breathing

Box breathing is a simple and effective stress management technique that involves breathing in a structured manner. The method is named for the four equal parts or "sides" of the breath cycle, similar to the sides of a box. Here is how it works:

1. **Inhale:** Slowly breathe in through your nose for a count of four seconds.

2. **Hold:** Hold your breath for a count of four seconds.

3. **Exhale:** Slowly breathe out through your mouth for a count of four seconds.

4. **Hold:** Hold your breath again for a count of four seconds.

Then, repeat the cycle as needed. This technique helps to calm the nervous system, increase focus, and reduce stress. It's commonly used by Navy SEALs, athletes, and individuals in high-stress professions, but it can be beneficial for anyone looking to manage stress and anxiety.

Box breathing can effectively bring your breaths per minute down to 3.75 breaths per minute. Here's the breakdown:

Each full cycle of box breathing (inhale, hold, exhale, hold) takes 16 seconds (4 seconds for each phase). There are 60 seconds in a minute, so:

Breaths per minute=60 seconds16 seconds per breath cycle=3.75 breaths per minuteBreaths per minute=16 seconds per breath cycle60 seconds=3.75 breaths per minute

This slower breathing rate helps activate the parasympathetic nervous system, promoting relaxation and reducing stress.

Box breathing impacts the body physiologically in several beneficial ways during each of its four phases:

1. **Inhale (4 seconds):**

   o **Physiological Impact:** During inhalation, the diaphragm contracts and moves downward, allowing the lungs to expand and fill with air. This increases the oxygen levels in the blood.

   o **Nervous System Response:** The act of deep, controlled inhalation stimulates the vagus nerve, which is part of the parasympathetic nervous system. This can help reduce the heart rate and promote a state of calmness.

2. **Hold (4 seconds):**

- **Physiological Impact:** Holding the breath allows for oxygen to diffuse from the alveoli in the lungs into the bloodstream more effectively, increasing oxygen saturation.

- **Nervous System Response:** This phase helps to balance oxygen and carbon dioxide levels in the blood, and the temporary pause can enhance mental focus and clarity by giving a brief moment of stillness.

3. **Exhale (4 seconds):**

- **Physiological Impact:** Exhalation involves the diaphragm relaxing and moving upward, pushing air out of the lungs and expelling carbon dioxide from the body.

- **Nervous System Response:** Slow and controlled exhalation is crucial for activating the parasympathetic nervous system. It helps to reduce heart rate, blood pressure, and stress hormone levels (like cortisol), contributing to a sense of relaxation and calmness.

4. **Hold (4 seconds):**

- **Physiological Impact:** The second holding phase allows the body to experience a momentary balance of having less oxygen and higher levels of carbon dioxide, which can stimulate a mild and beneficial stress response.

- **Nervous System Response:** This phase can help enhance resilience to stress by training the body to remain calm in situations where oxygen levels are lower, thereby improving overall stress tolerance and emotional regulation.

Overall, box breathing helps to regulate the autonomic nervous system, reducing the dominance of the sympathetic nervous system (associated with the fight-or-flight response) and enhancing the parasympathetic nervous system (associated with rest and digest). This balanced state can lead to improved mental clarity, reduced anxiety, and better overall physiological functioning.

The "Box" Pattern

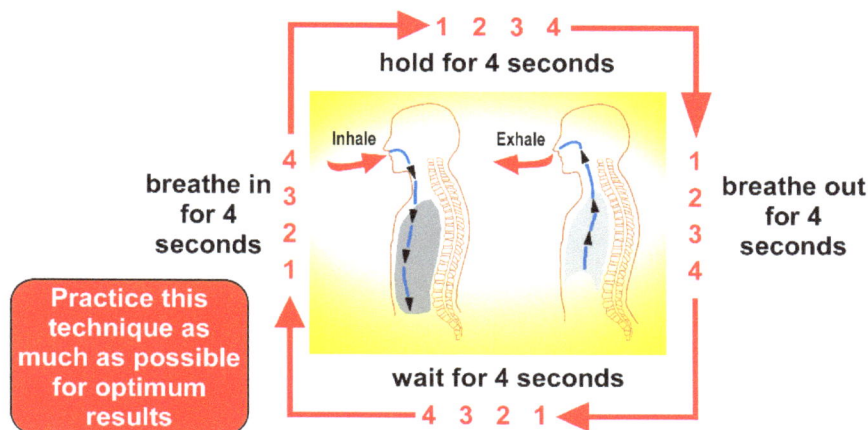

© Copyright 2023 - CAD Graphics, Inc.

Tibetan medicine seeks to draw attention to the relationship in balancing aspects of the mind, body, and behavior. Meditation is an integral component within Tibetan medicine. Through practices of Tibetan meditation, the practitioner seeks to probe the nature of reality. There is an emphasis to tame the incessant inner dialogue of our thoughts, which is constantly shifting to the barrage of sensory input. This inner dialogue is often referred to as the "monkey mind". Through these meditation methods one can transform the mind into a conduit to create better health and happiness (University of Minnesota, 2020).

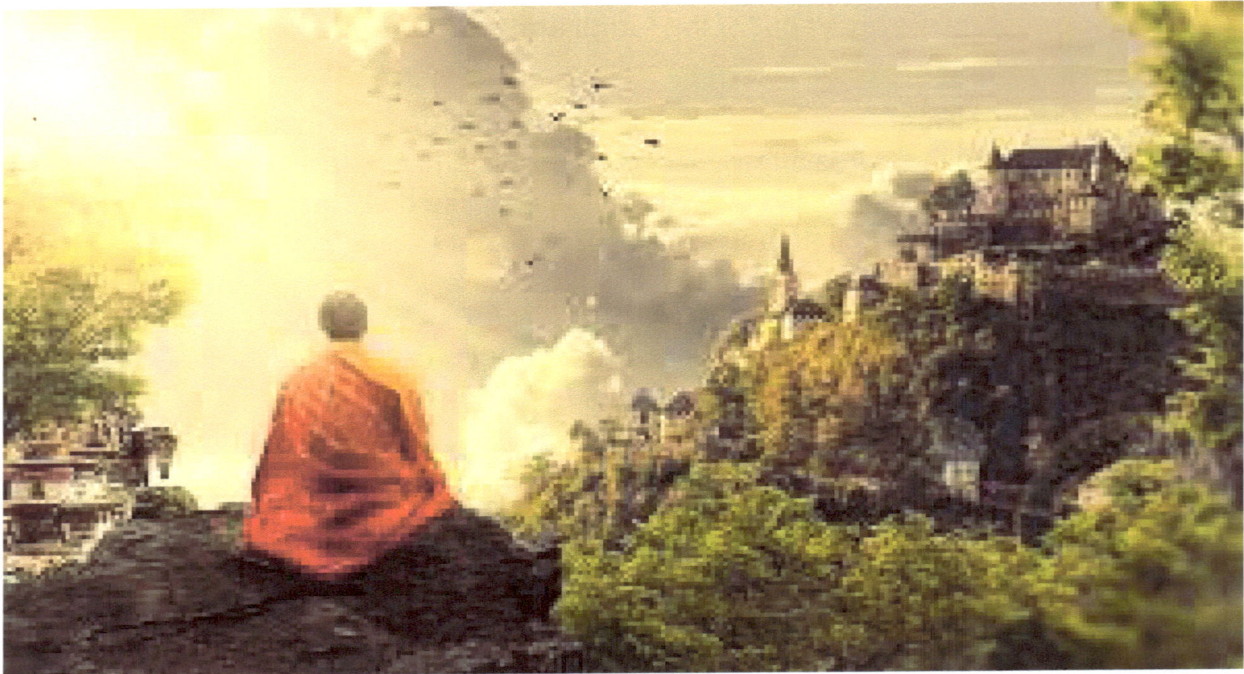

The ultimate goal of Buddhism is to reach *nirvana* or spiritual enlightenment where there is an absence of suffering or realization of the self and its relation to the universe.

Nirvana translates to "cessation", as in removing suffering and its undesired effects of drama, manipulation, aggression, struggle, etc. Practice of Tibetan meditation is a means that can lead to this goal.

Within Buddhism is the concept of The *Four Noble Truths*, which are relative to the meditation practices. These truths would be:

1. **Life is painful and frustrating**. Everyone experiences painful and frustrating moments.

2. **Suffering has a cause**. The cause comes from our attachment to what we know and is familiar.

3. **The cause of suffering can be ended by releasing expectations and attachments**. Attachment based on fear of loss and fear of being alone and separate are the causes of suffering.

4. **Meditation, or the practice of mindfulness and awareness, is the way to end suffering**

We can stop dwelling in the past by being focused on the current moment. Keeping these concepts at the forefront of our thoughts, will help with detachment and concentration, and lead to mastery of the mind (Yugay, 2018).

Sitting while meditating is a major component of Tibetan Meditation, I think it is important to note that these practices are more of a lifestyle where these truths are experienced and addressed throughout the whole day, every day, for the practitioner and not just something to ponder once in a while when it is convenient.

I found some information about the Dalai Lama that I found quite interesting. The Dalai Lama actually has his own website! Amazing how he has embraced modern technologies to further spread his teachings of awareness of compassion, suffering and other aspects of Buddhism and Tibetan Meditation. The Dalia Lama is the head monk of Tibetan Buddhism. His meditation schedule is a large portion of his daily routine, being quite intense compared to most people who meditate. He starts his days with a few hours of prayers, meditation, and prostration. After breakfast, he spends another three hours on meditation and prayer. After his 5 p.m. tea, the Dalai Lama concludes his day with another two more hours of meditation and then finishes with his evening prayers. Every day he spends about seven hours a day on mindfulness. He shares that even if you only commit five minutes a day to meditation, one can still gain the benefits of slowing aging, sharpening the mind, and reducing stress.

References:

6 Tips for Longevity From the Dalai Lama | Well+Good (wellandgood.com)Links to an external site.

His Holiness the 14th Dalai Lama | The 14th Dalai Lama

University of Minnesota. (2020, May). *How Can I Practice Tibetan Meditation?* https://www.takingcharge.csh.umn.edu/how-can-i-practice-tibetan-meditationLinks to an external site.

Yugay, I. (2018, January 19). *The Secret To Enlightenment With Buddhist Meditation*. Mindvalley. https://blog.mindvalley.com/buddhist-meditation/Links to an external site.

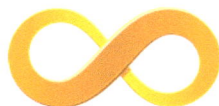

Across time and cultures, the greatest spiritual teachers have emphasized simplicity, humility, and inner transformation. Yet, paradoxically, the institutions that grow around these teachings often accumulate material wealth, political power, and ego-driven prestige.

Christianity, Buddhism, Hinduism, Islam, all at their core, advocate for the shedding of worldly attachments. Yet many of their largest institutions exhibit the very materialism and hierarchy their founders warned against. In light of today's cultural unrest, consumerism, and spiritual seeking, these contradictions deserve closer reflection.

A Humble Beginning

Jesus of Nazareth lived with radical humility. His birth in a manger (Luke 2:7, New International Version [NIV]), his itinerant lifestyle (*"the Son of Man has no place to lay his head,"* Luke 9:58, NIV), and his repeated critiques of religious legalism (Matthew 23:1–28, NIV) demonstrate a clear rejection of material power and ritualized pretense.

He warned against storing up treasures on earth, urging people instead to seek spiritual treasures (Matthew 6:19–21, NIV). His message was direct: inner transformation and compassion mattered more than public ritual or personal gain.

And yet, centuries later, the Roman Catholic Church emerged from the very empire that crucified him, to became one of the wealthiest and most ritualized institutions in human history (MacCulloch, 2011).

A Universal Paradox

This irony is not exclusive to Christianity. It is a universal pattern across major belief systems:

- **Buddhism**: Siddhartha Gautama, the Buddha, renounced his royal status to seek enlightenment through simplicity and meditation. His core teaching of the elimination of craving and attachment became institutionalized into monasteries and sects, some of which, over centuries, accumulated wealth, political influence, and hierarchical authority (Lopez, 2001).

- **Hinduism**: Early Vedic teachings stressed detachment from material life through paths like *Jnana* (knowledge) and *Bhakti* (devotion). Yet, sprawling temple complexes, priestly hierarchies, and caste structures often mirrored societal materialism and status-seeking (Flood, 1996).

- **Islam**: The Prophet Muhammad lived simply, called for humility, and emphasized equality among believers. Yet throughout history, caliphates and modern regimes alike have at times entangled faith with vast political and material ambitions (Esposito, 1998).

Again and again, humanity seems to be drawn to codify spiritual simplicity into worldly complexity.

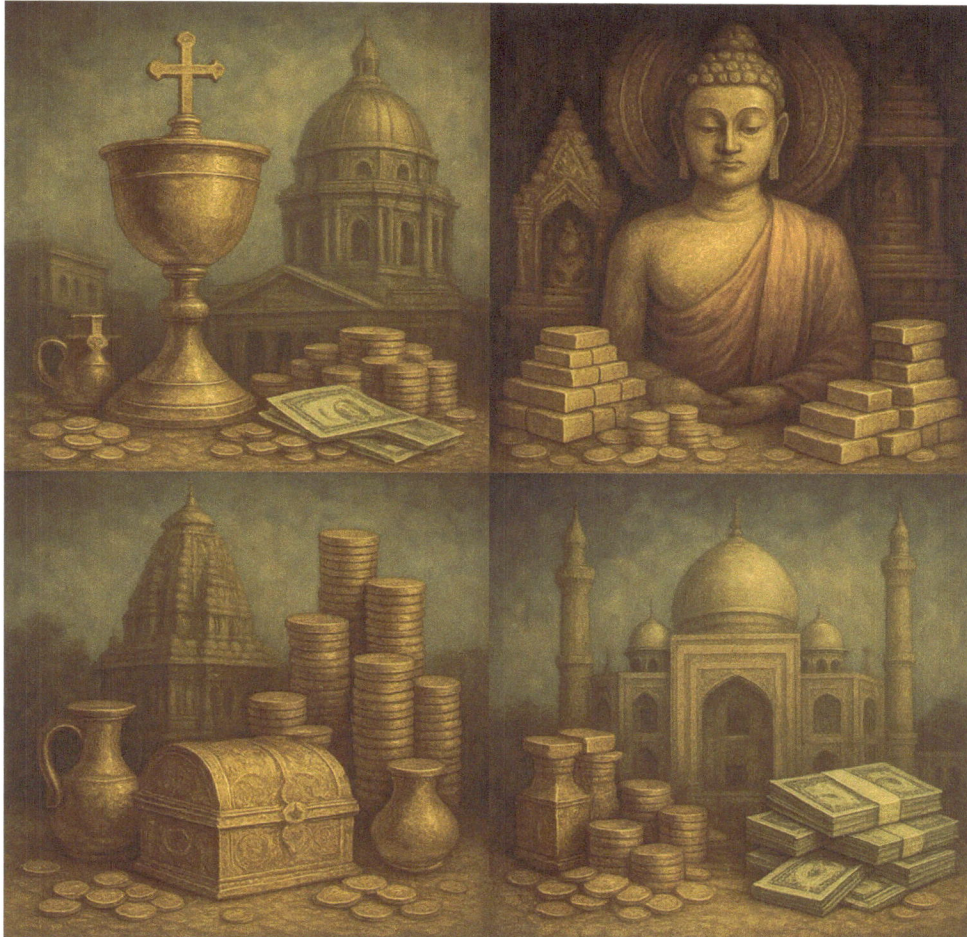

Why Does This Happen?

From a psychological and sociological standpoint, this paradox might stem from natural human tendencies:

- **Desire for Security**: Spiritual communities often accumulate resources to protect their teachings and communities from external threats.

- **Institutionalization**: Movements grow into organizations, and organizations seek stability, leading to bureaucracy and hierarchy.

- **Human Ego**: Even with the best intentions, individuals and groups may seek recognition, authority, and influence, contradicting the original teachings.

As the Tao Te Ching observes, *"The higher the structure, the farther from the Way"* (Laozi, trans. Mitchell, 1988).

Cultural Relevance Today

Today's society, riddled with consumerism, curated self-images, and institutional distrust, mirrors these spiritual paradoxes. Many seekers are disillusioned with religious structures not because they reject faith, but because they crave *authenticity*.

Holistic health practitioners recognize that wellness is found in true balance of mind, body, and spirit, and requires stripping away external noise and realigning with essential truths. It's not in grandeur but in simplicity that healing often occurs.

The example of figures like Jesus, Buddha, and Muhammad calls us back not to ritualized identity, but to the living essence of humility, compassion, and conscious living.

A Personal Reflection

This reflection isn't a condemnation of all spiritual institutions. Rather, it is a call to vigilance:

- Are we aligning with the heart of spiritual wisdom or merely its outer forms?
- Are we living simply, authentically, and compassionately, or becoming entangled in ego, status, and recognition?

As individuals seeking holistic well-being, we are invited to live in *the spirit* rather than merely follow *the form*.

Spiritual maturity requires discernment and choosing the inward journey over external display, whether in religion, health, or daily life.

References:

Esposito, J. L. (1998). *Islam: The straight path* (3rd ed.). Oxford University Press.

Flood, G. (1996). *An introduction to Hinduism*. Cambridge University Press.

Lopez, D. S., Jr. (2001). *THE STORY OF BUDDHISM*. HarperSanFrancisco. http://www.chanreads.org/wp-content/uploads/2022/09/The-Story-of-Buddhism-A-Concise-Guide-to-Its-History-Teachings-Donald-S.-Lopez-Jr.-chanreads.org_.pdf

MacCulloch, D. (2011). *Christianity: The first three thousand years*. Penguin Books.
Mitchell, S. (Trans.). (1988). *Tao Te Ching* (Lao Tzu). Harper & Row.

The Holy Bible, New International Version. (2011). Biblica, Inc. (Original work published 1978)

SECTION VII: NEUROLOGY, SENSORY SYSTEMS & AWARENESS

A Holistic Guide to Interoception, Exteroception, and Proprioception

In the world of holistic health, awareness is everything. Cultivating mindfulness and tuning into both the body and the environment are foundational to wellness. But did you know that your body has specialized ways of sensing the world *within* and *around* you? Also, not just through the classic five senses, but through internal systems of perception that guide how you feel, move, and connect with life.

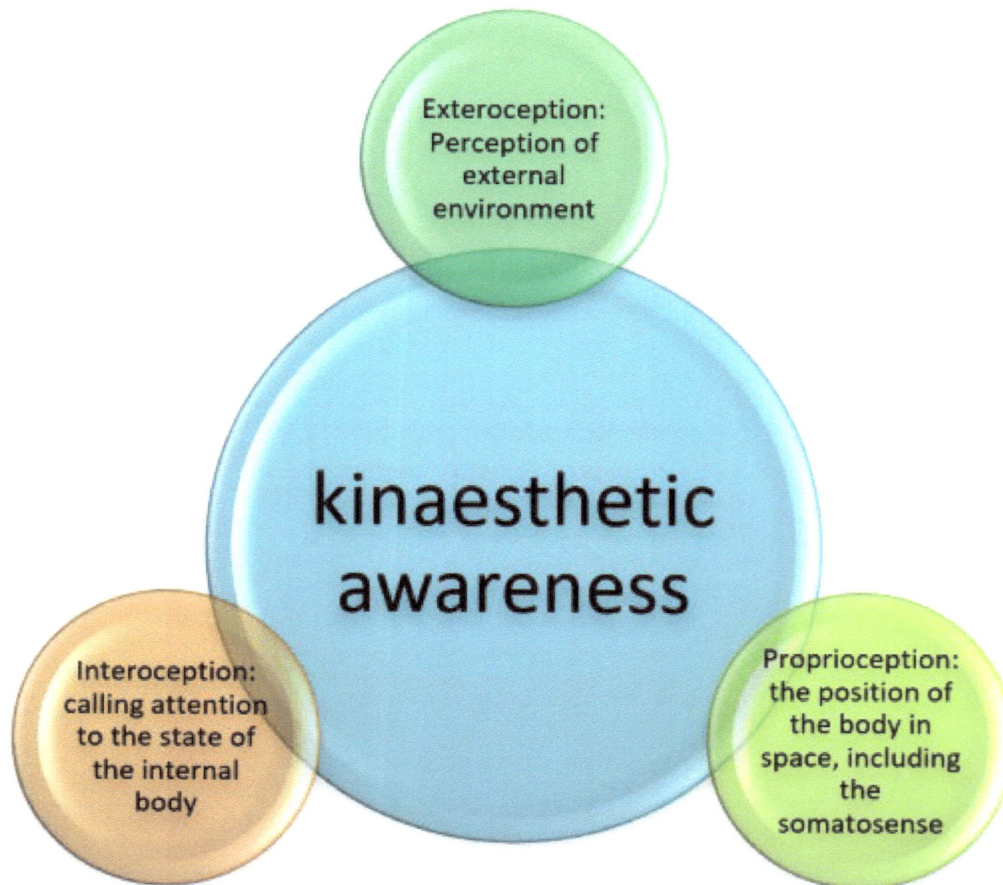

Let's explore three vital sensory systems that shape our well-being: **interoception**, **exteroception**, and **proprioception**—along with **kinesthesia**, a close ally in movement awareness.

Interoception: Listening to the Body's Inner Language

Interoception is your body's ability to sense what's happening inside. It's how you know when you're hungry, thirsty, full, tired, or anxious. It's the feeling of your heart pounding during stress, or the warmth of calm spreading through your chest after deep breathing.

Wellness Tip: Enhancing interoception through practices like breathwork, mindful eating, or body scans can improve emotional regulation, reduce anxiety, and deepen your self-awareness.

Exteroception: Engaging with the Outside World

This is your ability to sense the external environment through sight, sound, smell, touch, and taste. It's how you hear music, feel the breeze on your skin, or taste your morning tea.

Wellness Tip: Mindful sensory experiences such as walking barefoot in nature or savoring a meal, can ground you in the present and relieve overstimulation from digital overload.

Proprioception: Knowing Where You Are in Space

Proprioception is your sense of body position and movement without needing to look. It lets you touch your nose with eyes closed or maintain balance on one foot.

Wellness Tip: Proprioception is sharpened through methods such as yoga, tai chi, martial arts, and balance exercises. It's essential for preventing falls, improving posture, and developing fluid movement.

Kinesthesia: The Sense of Movement

Closely related to proprioception, kinesthesia is your ability to sense the motion of your body parts. While proprioception tells you where your limbs *are*, kinesthesia tells you how they're *moving*. It's the awareness that lets dancers glide, athletes react, and everyday movements flow with grace.

Wellness Tip: Kinesthetic awareness grows through conscious movement with practices like qigong, dance, or somatic movement therapy awaken this sense and re-pattern the nervous system for ease and flow.

Why This Matters in Modern Life

In today's fast-paced world, many people are "cut off" from their bodies and living mostly in their heads, overwhelmed by information, and physically stagnant. Reconnecting with these sensory systems isn't just about moving better; it's about *living better*.

- **Interoception** helps us feel more emotionally in tune.

- **Exteroception** draws us into the richness of the moment.

- **Proprioception** keeps us balanced and safe.

- **Kinesthesia** invites freedom and fluidity into our movement.

When we train these senses through stillness, movement, reflection, and sensation we reclaim our full human experience.
Wellness is not just about what we do, but about how deeply we sense and experience ourselves while doing it. By developing these subtle yet powerful senses, we become more grounded, responsive, and resilient—physically, mentally, and spiritually.

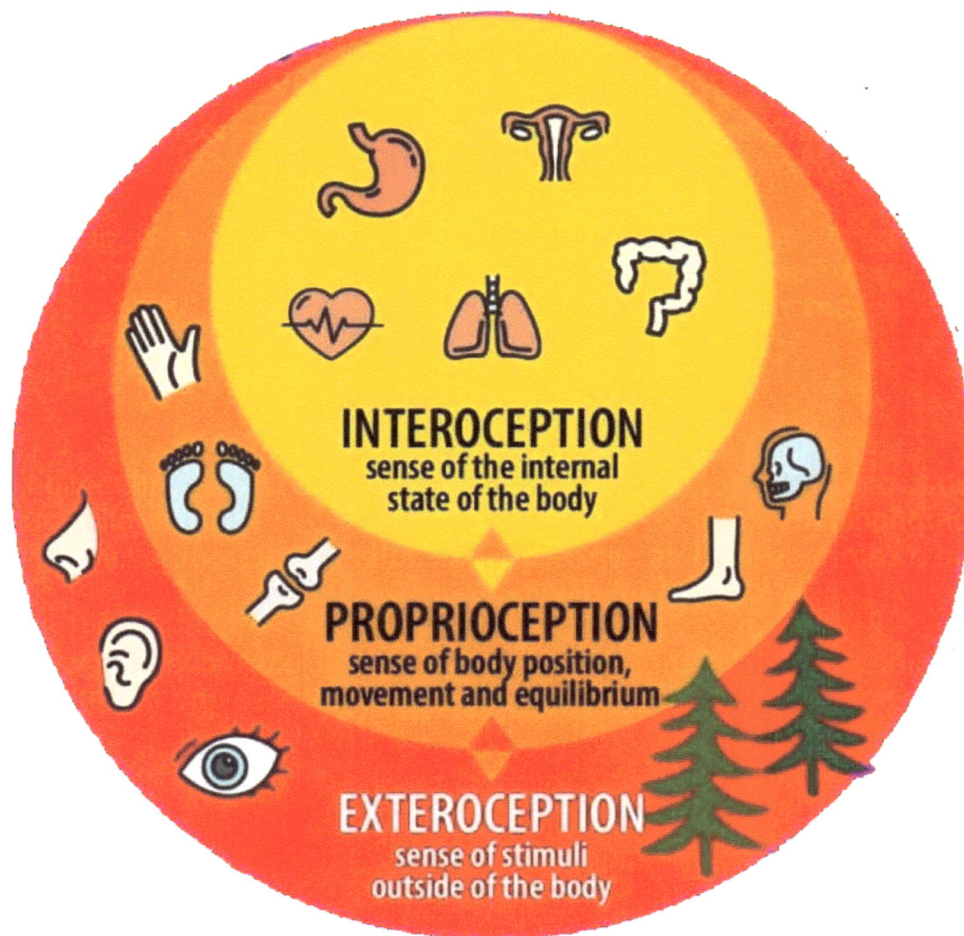

INTEROCEPTION
sense of the internal
state of the body

PROPRIOCEPTION
sense of body position,
movement and equilibrium

EXTEROCEPTION
sense of stimuli
outside of the body

In the realm of holistic wellness, we often focus on diet, exercise, breath, and mindset, but how often do we consider our *ears* and our sense of balance as essential tools for mental clarity and cognitive performance?

Dr. Andrew Huberman, a Stanford neuroscientist and host of the *Huberman Lab Podcast,* explores this overlooked territory in his episode *"How Hearing & Balance Enhance Focus & Learning."* As someone deeply invested in integrating modern science with ancient wellness practices, I found this episode not only affirming but eye-opening. Let me break down some of the most practical insights.

The Auditory System: A Biological Prism for the Mind

Huberman explains the auditory system in great detail: how the outer ear captures sound waves, how the eardrum passes those vibrations through three tiny bones (malleus, incus, stapes), and how the cochlea, which is the fluid-filled spiral in the inner ear, transforms those vibrations into neural signals.

What stood out was the *prism-like function* of the cochlea. Much like a prism that separates light into colors, the cochlea separates sound into different frequencies. This allows the brain to decipher complex soundscapes like music, voices, and environmental cues. For those of us practicing mindfulness, this gives new meaning to the phrase *"intentional listening."*

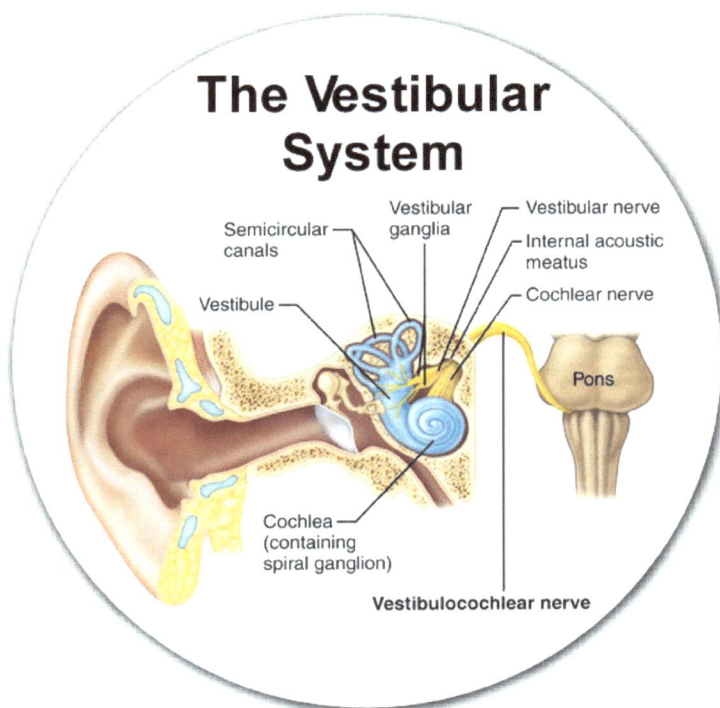

150

Binaural Beats: Sound as a Mental Tuning Fork

Huberman dives into the use of *binaural beats*, where two slightly different frequencies are played in each ear. The brain interprets the difference as a single beat, which can influence brainwave activity. He shares that binaural beats can help promote states such as focus (beta waves), calm (alpha), and deep meditation (theta). While not a cure-all, they are a valuable tool, especially when integrated with practices like breathwork, yoga, or qigong.

- **Delta and Theta**: Sleep and deep meditation
- **Alpha**: Calm focus
- **Beta**: Alertness
- **Gamma**: Heightened cognition and insight

White Noise: A Double-Edged Sword

Surprisingly, Huberman discusses how *low-level white noise* can actually enhance learning and motivation. It does this by increasing dopamine release, which is our brain's reward chemical. This may explain why many people, me included, prefer ambient noise while working or studying.

However, there's a cautionary note: prolonged white noise exposure in infants may hinder healthy auditory development. White noise lacks the variation necessary to develop *tonotopic maps, which are t*he brain's way of organizing sound frequencies. In short, while useful for adults, white noise can be detrimental if misused during critical developmental windows in children.

The Cocktail Party Effect: Cognitive Load in Action

Another fascinating point is the *cocktail party effect,* where the brain's ability to focus on a single voice (selective awareness) in a noisy room. Huberman emphasizes how much effort this takes. It's a reminder that modern life, full of overlapping stimuli, can tax our nervous system in subtle but real ways. As holistic practitioners, this reinforces the importance of quiet time, sound baths, and low-stimulation environments to support mental clarity.

Balance and the Vestibular System: Movement as Medicine

Perhaps the most profound yet underappreciated insight from Dr. Huberman's episode is the role of the *vestibular system*. This is the sensory network within the inner ear that helps detect head orientation and movement. Though commonly associated with balance, this system is directly linked to emotional regulation, attention, and brain flexibility.
When we engage in movements that challenge balance, like skateboarding, walking on uneven terrain, or even standing on one leg with eyes closed, we activate the semicircular canals and otolith organs that send signals to the brainstem about head motion and

gravitational shifts. These inputs, in turn, stimulate the release of dopamine and serotonin, the neurochemicals responsible for motivation, well-being, and neuroplasticity (Huberman, 2025).

Why This Matters:

- **Dopamine** fuels focus, drive, and memory encoding.
- **Serotonin** calms the nervous system and stabilizes mood.

Vestibular engagement stimulates these systems through subtle head movements and changes in posture. Simple activities such as:

- Balancing with eyes closed,
- Turning the head during walking,
- Forward-accelerating sports like biking or skating,
- Practicing head tilts during yoga, qigong, tai chi and other martial arts

These activities can elevate mood and sharpen learning by improving sensory-motor integration and activating brain regions like the locus coeruleus and ventral tegmental area (VTA), critical dopamine centers (Hitier et al., 2014).

From a holistic point of view, these effects mirror what Eastern disciplines have long known that physical movement, balance, and breath are gateways to emotional equilibrium and mental clarity. By training the vestibular system regularly, we condition the brain to stay agile, focused, and resilient under pressure.

Dynamic Exercises to Improve Your Sense of Balance

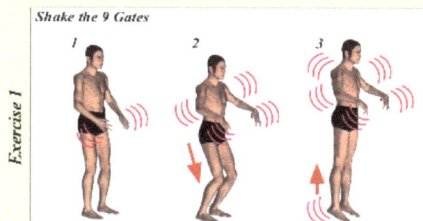

Exercise 1 — Shake the 9 Gates
NOTES: 1- Loosely shake hands & fingers. 2- Continue shaking hands working your way up to elbows & shoulders. Bend & straighten knees while shaking upper body. 3- Same motion but add gentle bouncing forward on to the balls of the feet.

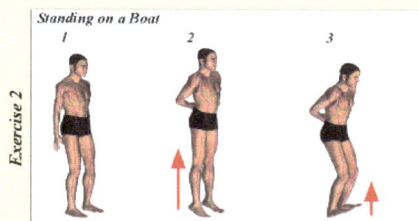

Exercise 2 — Standing on a Boat
NOTES: 1-Inhale as arching the lower back. 2- Rock forward onto the balls of the feet. 3- Exhale as rocking back onto the heels, while tucking the tailbone slightly forward.

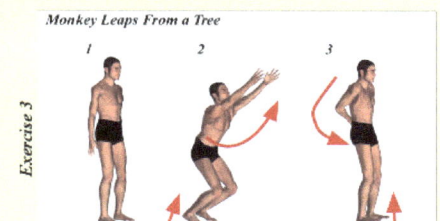

Exercise 3 — Monkey Leaps From a Tree
NOTES: 1- Start in a neutral position. 2- Inhale as swinging arms forward, rock on to balls of feet. 3- Exhale while bringing hands to lower back, round back & tuck tailbone forward, rock on to heels.

www.MindandBodyExercises.com   (c) Copyright 2021 - CAD Graphics, Inc.

Body Components Connected to Balance

Brain
The brain processes the signals from the eyes, inner ear and the sensory systems (skin, joints, muscles, nerves) of the human body.

Eyes
The eyes relate information to the brain such as spatial orientation and environmental conditions.

Muscles
The muscular system provides strength and stability to the skeletal systems, while maintaining flexibility in movement.

Joints
Healthy joints help form a strong foundation for the body to navigate daily activities. Vibrations in movement are transferred through the bones and muscles to the brain to process.

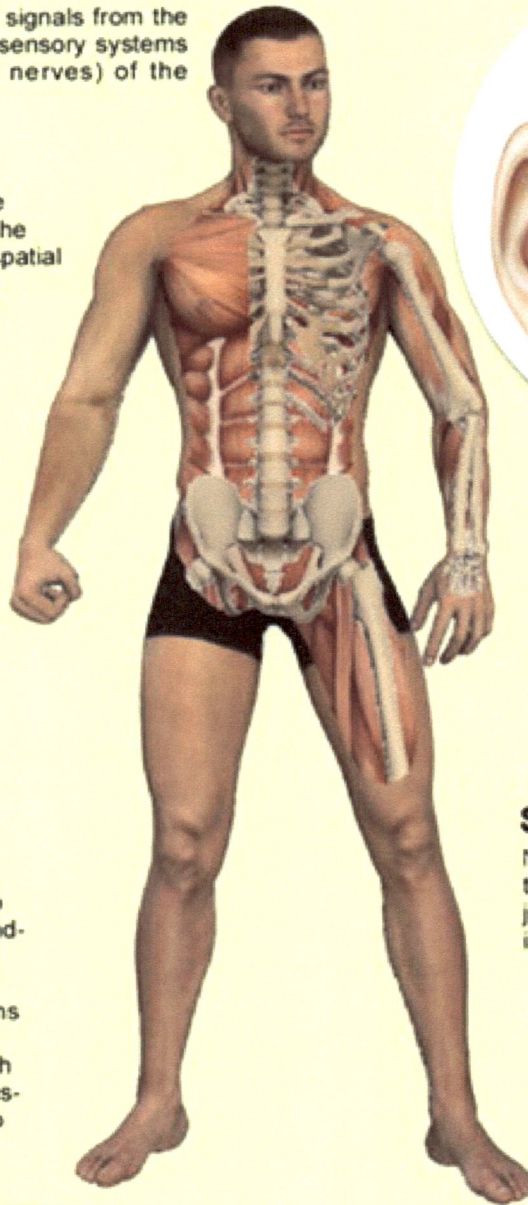

The Vestibular System

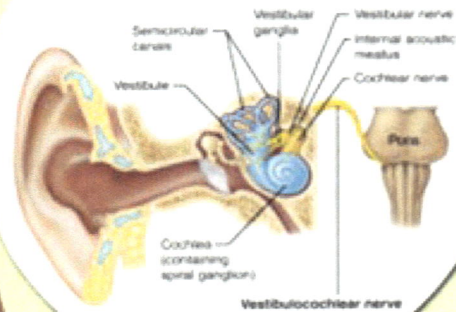

Inner ear
The inner ear and the Vestibular system, regulates equilibrium while providing directional information to the brain to process.

Sensory Receptors
Nerves in the joints called proprioceptors, sense vibrations that flow through joints, muscles and skin sending the information to the brain to process.

Vestibular-ocular Reflex

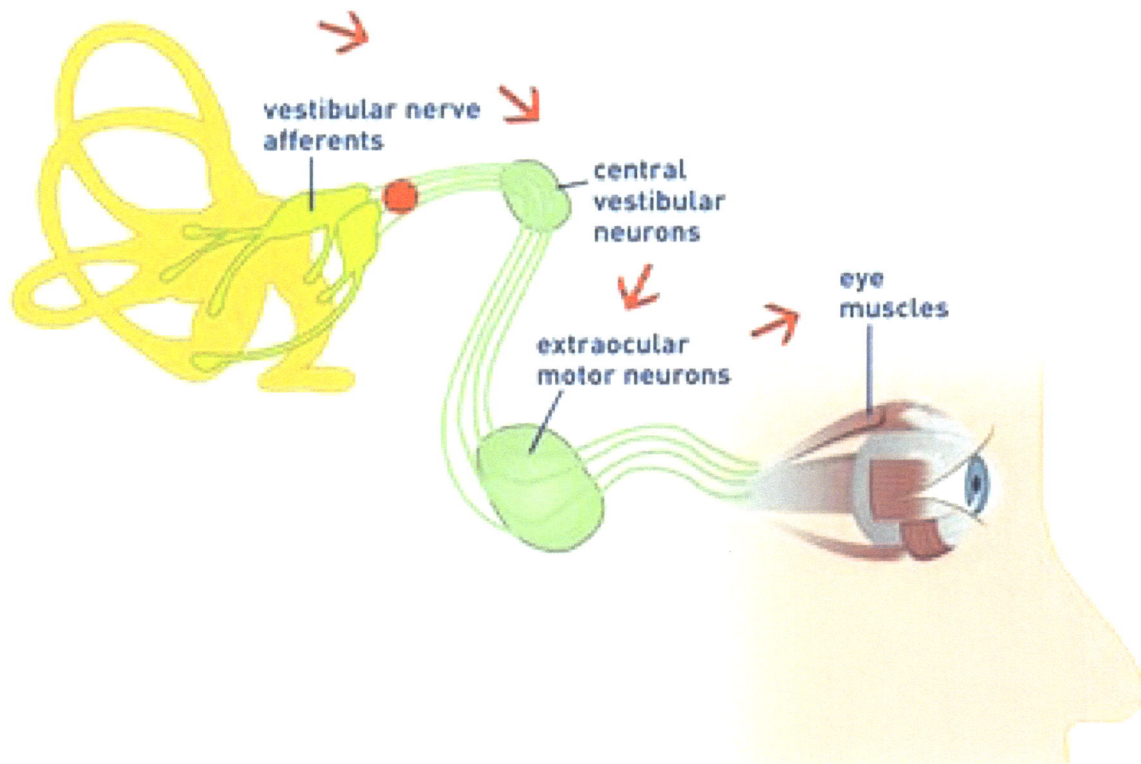

vestibular nerve afferents

central vestibular neurons

extraocular motor neurons

eye muscles

Holistic Takeaways: Harmonizing the Senses

Dr. Huberman's breakdown of the hearing and balance systems mirrors much of what traditional holistic systems have long emphasized: sensitivity, movement, and sensory integration are keys to mental clarity. As a practitioner and educator of mind-body methods, I see incredible value in integrating these insights:

- Use **binaural beats** or ambient nature sounds during meditation or study sessions.

- Encourage balance training as part of daily physical routines with eyes-closed stance work, walking meditation (Tai Chi, Qigong, BaguaZhang), or even play-based movement.

- Be mindful of auditory overload in modern environments. Sometimes, the most powerful medicine is silence.

Final Thoughts

In holistic health, we strive for integration of not just the body, mind, and spirit, but also of physiological systems that we often take for granted. Dr. Huberman's insights into hearing and balance affirm that our senses are not passive. They are gateways to enhanced learning, mood regulation, and cognitive vitality.

By engaging in the auditory and vestibular systems intentionally, we can improve not just our ability to hear or stand upright but to learn, grow, and live with greater awareness.

References:

Huberman, A. (2025, May 8). *How hearing & balance enhance focus & learning*. YouTube. https://www.youtube.com/watch?v=fSBgDq2ttCw

Hitier, M., Besnard, S., & Smith, P. F. (2014). Vestibular pathways involved in cognition. *Frontiers in Integrative Neuroscience*, 8, 59. https://doi.org/10.3389/fnint.2014.00059

Lopez, C., Blanke, O., & Mast, F. W. (2012). The human vestibular cortex revealed by coordinate-based meta-analysis. *Neuroscience*, 212, 159–179. https://doi.org/10.1016/j.neuroscience.2012.03.028

Smith, P. F., & Zheng, Y. (2013). From ear to uncertainty: vestibular contributions to cognitive function. *Frontiers in Integrative Neuroscience*, 7. https://doi.org/10.3389/fnint.2013.00084

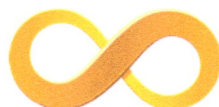

What is Health?

"Health is more than the absence of disease symptoms. The true goal is sustainable balance, as recognized by chiropractors and other holistically oriented health practitioners."

Micozzi, Marc S.. Fundamentals of Complementary, Alternative, and Integrative Medicine – E-Book (p. 544). Elsevier Health Sciences. Kindle Edition.

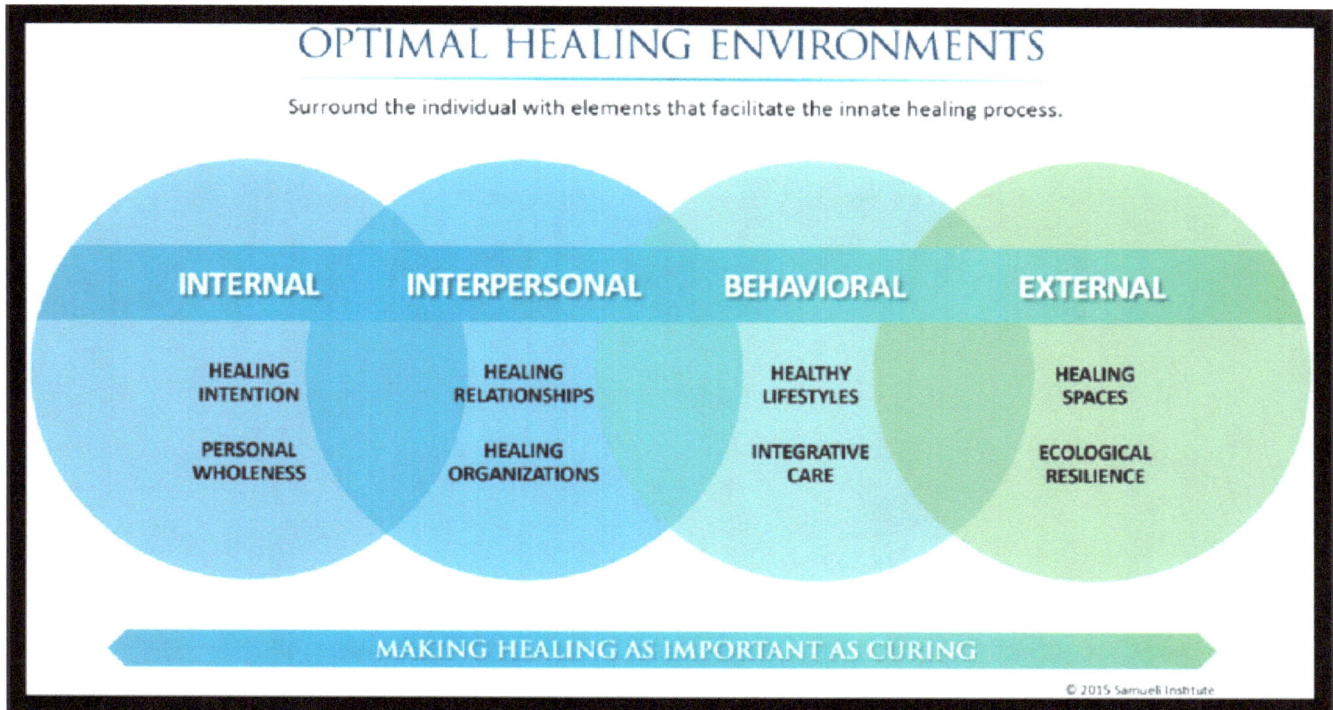

"The low-grade viral or fungal infections, the persistent catarrhal state, recurrent headaches or migraines, allergies, skin and arthritic disease and other chronic inflammatory diseases, stress problems and anxiety neuroses and cancer are all marked by a failure to cope or adequately to defend. One perspective on this development is that modern medicine has so effectively neutered the acute disease, especially in the too frequent use of antibiotics and anti-inflammatories, that most people in developed countries have never had to muster their defenses. Life is also much easier in these societies and there is generally less rigorous testing of physiological functions."

Bone, Kerry; Mills, Simon. Principles and Practice of Phytotherapy (p. 85). Elsevier Health Sciences. Kindle Edition.

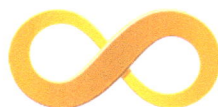

Excerpt from: Principles and Practice of Phytotherapy, by Kerry Bone

Convalescence

It is notable that at the time when healthcare has to address numerous chronic and debilitating diseases, it has moved away from traditional strategic approaches. Historically, a period of recovery after illness was considered essential to prevent recurrence. Convalescent care was once the primary treatment for severe diseases, exemplified by European sanatoria for tuberculosis patients.

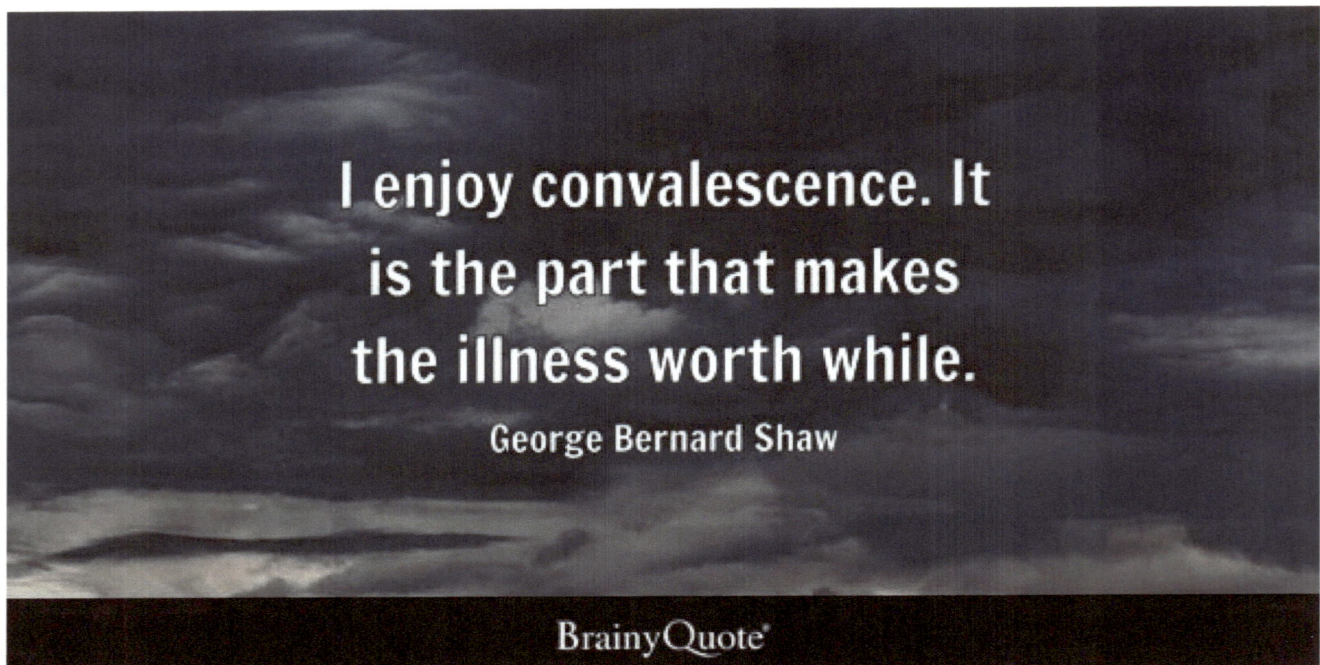

I enjoy convalescence. It is the part that makes the illness worth while.

George Bernard Shaw

BrainyQuote

The practice of convalescence diminished as modern drugs like penicillin and steroid anti-inflammatories provided rapid resolution of diseases, including tuberculosis. As healthcare provision improved and public expectations grew, hospital stays became shorter, and the demands of modern life led people to forgo convalescence after illnesses such as flu, increasing the likelihood of recurrence.

Effective convalescence enhances recovery, strengthens immune defenses, and provides protection against recurrence. It is crucial for recovering from debilitating diseases, fatigue syndromes, recurrent infections, and states of compromised immunity. Convalescence requires time, which is increasingly difficult to find.

There are four essential features of convalescence:

Rest

Rest is the most important element, including maximum sleep, as this is the body's time for repair. In early stages, constant sleep should be encouraged, followed by promoting rest as much as possible. Rest also means reduced activity: work should be done in short bursts, switching frequently between tasks. Patients should pace themselves, prioritize sleep, and avoid unnecessary work. Mental rest is paramount: sleep takes precedence over other activities.

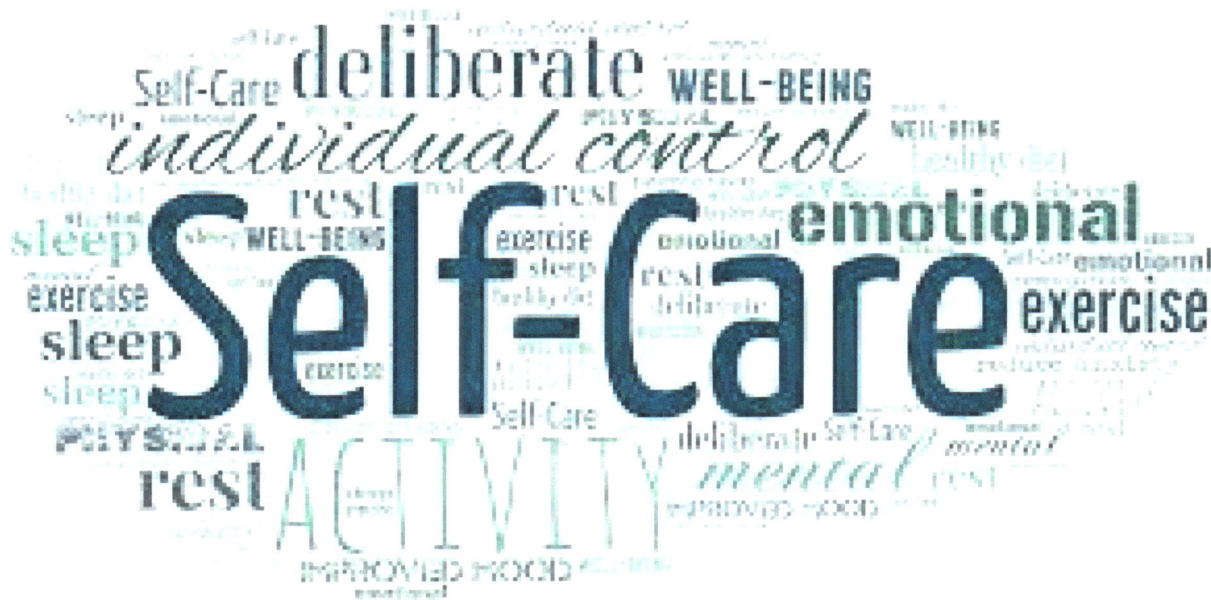

Exercise

Exercise complements rest and prevents congestion and stagnation. The body needs brief daily aerobic exercise, defined as any activity producing a pulse rate of 60–80% of 220 minus one's age. Using pulse rate to set exercise levels is self-adjusting; debilitated individuals reach high pulse rates with minimal activity. Exercise should not cause more fatigue. Building up to 15 minutes of aerobic activity daily dissipates sympathetic-adrenergic effects and encourages better sleep.

Diet

A convalescent diet should nourish without stimulating or imposing demands. Based on vegetables, cereals, pulses, fish, eggs, chicken, and fowl, it excludes stimulants, caffeine, nicotine, alcohol, sugar, dairy food, convenience foods, and additives. A simple peasant diet, respecting food and incorporating it into daily rhythms, is recommended.

Medication

Maintaining treatment during convalescence is important, whether herbal or conventional. Herbal remedies can facilitate recovery when rest, exercise, and diet alone is insufficient. Remedies may include warming herbs for febrile disease recovery and immune-supporting herbs for chronic infections. Digestive support and gentle cleansing are also necessary.

Phytotherapists often use convalescence to address chronic debilitated conditions such as fatigue syndrome or persistent infections. Many problems begin with an early-life infection. Completing convalescence from the original illness may be suggested, using appropriate remedies.

Bone, Kerry; Mills, Simon. Principles and Practice of Phytotherapy (pp. 86-87). Elsevier Health Sciences. Kindle Edition.

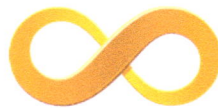

Glossary

Abdominal breathing – effective, diaphragmatic breathing that fills your lungs fully, reaches all the way down to your abdomen, slows your breathing rate, and helps you relax.

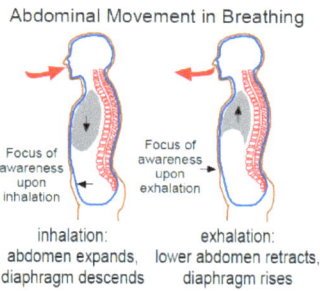

Abdominal Movement in Breathing

Focus of awareness upon inhalation

Focus of awareness upon exhalation

inhalation: abdomen expands, diaphragm descends

exhalation: lower abdomen retracts, diaphragm rises

Bagua (or Pa Kua) / 8-trigrams - eight symbols used in Daoist philosophy to represent the fundamental principles of reality, seen as a range of eight interrelated concepts. Each consists of three lines, each line either "broken" or "unbroken," respectively representing yin or yang.

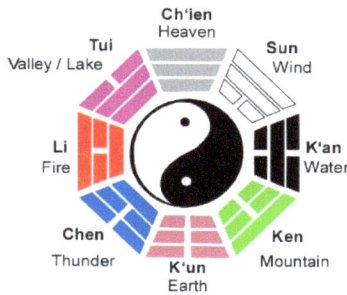

Ch'ien Heaven
Tui Valley / Lake
Sun Wind
Li Fire
K'an Water
Chen Thunder
K'un Earth
Ken Mountain

The Brass Basin – sits within the lower abdomen, touching at the navel in the front, between L2 & L3 vertebrae in the back and the perineum at the base.

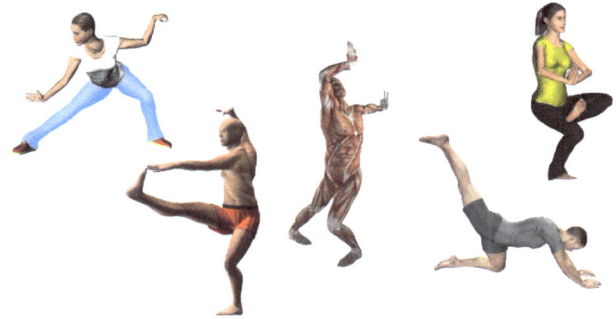

Mingmen-GV4 L2-L3, Gate of Life Kidney Point

Hui Yin-CV1 Meeting of Yin Gate of Life and Death Perineum

Qihai-CV6 Sea of Qi, Navel Point, Spleen

Bubbling Well - an energetic point located in the sole of the foot, slightly in front of the arch between the 2nd and 3rd toe. In the meridian system it is the same as the Kidney 1 point.

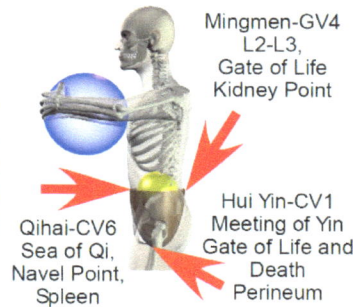

Kidney-1

Dan Tian - 3 energy centers Lower Dan Tian (1 of 3) - also known as the "sea of qi," is positioned below and behind the naval encompassing your lower bowl and is closely related to jing (or physical essence).

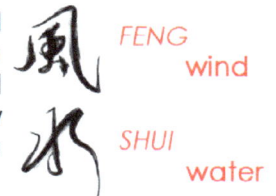

Shen-Spirit Upper Dantian (Field of Light)

Qi-Energy Middle Dantian (Field of Vibration)

Jing-Essence Lower Dantian (Field of Heat)

Daoyin, DaoYi, Daoist Yoga, Qigong – all names for energy exercises, with specific postures, little or no physical body movement and mindful regulated breathing patterns.

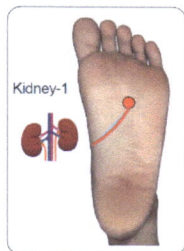

Feng Shui – translated into 'wind and water'; it is a Chinese philosophical system that teaches how to balance the energies in any given space.

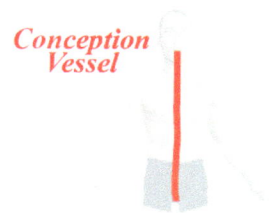

FENG wind

SHUI water

Conception Vessel (Ren Mai) – flows up the midline of the front of the body and governs all of the yin channels. The Conception Vessel is connected to the Thrusting and Yin Linking vessels.

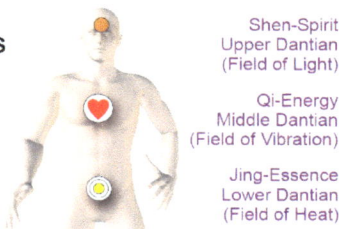

Conception Vessel

Governing Vessel (Du Mai) - flows up the midline of the back and governs all the Yang channels.

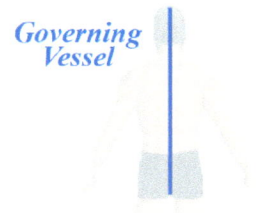

Governing Vessel

General Yu Fei – creator of the 8 Pieces of Brocade set.

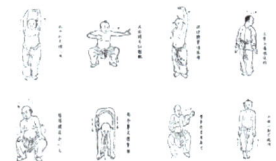

160

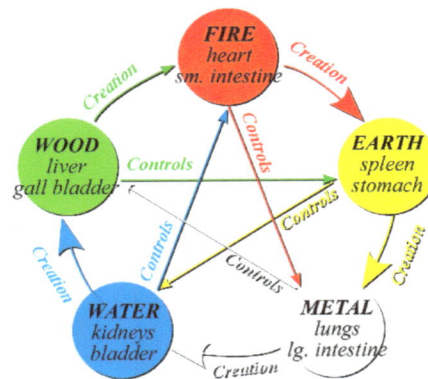

Controlling Cycle – the controlling or regulating sequence of the 5 element cycle. Wood controls Earth; Earth controls Water; Water controls Fire; Fire controls Metal; Metal controls Wood

Generating Cycle – the creative sequence of the 5 element cycle. Wood generates Fire; Fire generates Earth; Earth generates Metal; Metal generates Water; Water generates Wood.

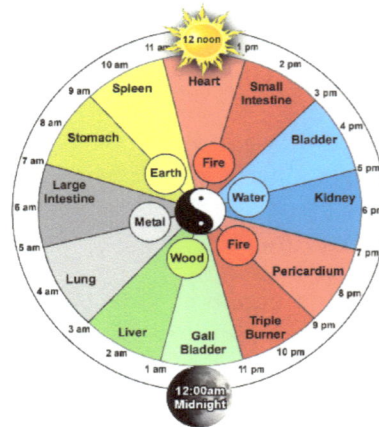

Horary Cycle - 24 Hour Qi Flow Though the Meridians; This cycle is known as the Horary cycle or the Circadian Clock. As Qi (energy) makes its way through the meridians, each meridian in turn with its associated organ, has a two-hour period during which it is at maximum energy.

Jing Well - The Jing (Well) points are 1 of 5 of The Five Element Points (shu) of the 12 energy meridians. They are located on the fingers and toes of the four extremities. These points are thought to be where the Qi of the meridians emerges and begins moving towards the trunk of the body. These are of upmost importance in that these points can help restore balance within the energy flow throughout the human body.

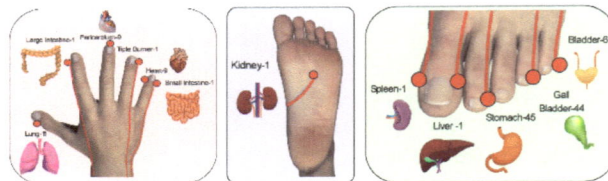

Meridians - a meridian is an 'energy highway' in the human body. There are 12 meridians and each is paired with an organ. Qi energy flows through these meridians or energy highways.

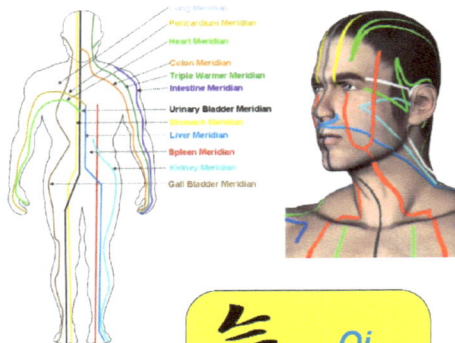

Qigong - or Chi Kung, is breathing exercises, with little or no body movement, that can adjust the brain waves to the Alpha state. When the mind is relaxed, the body chemistry changes and promotes natural healing.

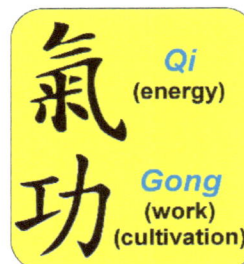

San Jiao (Triple Burner/Heater) – is a meridian line that regulates respiration, digestion and elimination. It is responsible for the movement and transformation of various solids and fluids throughout the system, as well as for the production and circulation of nourishing and protective energy.

Upper Burner	**WEI QI**
Middle Burner	**YING QI**
Lower Burner	**YUAN QI**

Nine Gates - the energy gates in your body are major relay stations where the strength of your Qi are regulated. These gates are located at joints or, more precisely, in the actual space between the bones of a joint. The nine gates are located at the shoulder, elbow and wrists, hip, knee and ankles, and along the cervical, the thoracic, and the lumbar spine.

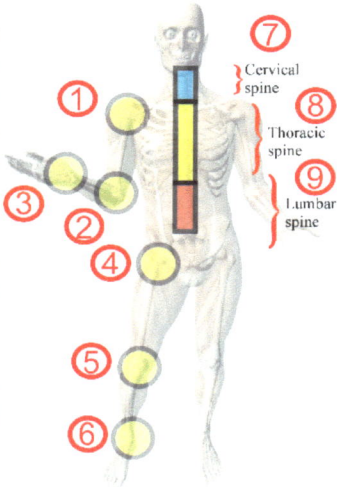

Three Treasures – Jing, Qi & Shen

Jing – (essence) the physical, yin and most dense of the Three Treasures. Think of Jing as a candle, specifically the quality and quantity of the wax.

Qi, chi or ki - (energy/breath) the energetic, vital force within all living things and it the most refined Treasure. Think of Qi as the burning flame of the candle.

Shen – (consciousness or spirit, is the most subtle of the Three Treasures and is the vitality behind Jing and Qi. Think of Shen as the light or illumination produced from the flame.

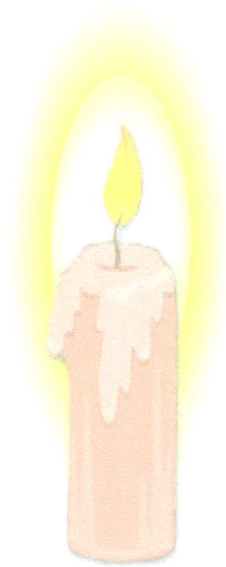

Seven Energy Centers – also known as chakras, are energy points in the subtle body that start at the base of the spinal column, continue through the sacral, solar plexus, heart, throat, eyebrow and end in the midst of the head vertex at the crown.

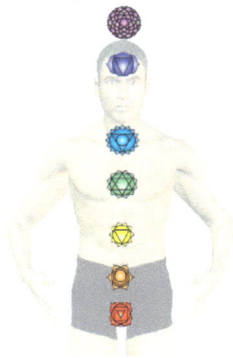

Six Healing Sounds – auditory sounds used for clearing internal (yin) organs and other tissues of stagnant Qi.

Metal - Hissss	Water - Chuuu	Wood - Shiiiii	Fire - Haaaa	Earth - Hoooo	6th Qi - Heeee
○	●	●	●	●	●
Lungs Lg. Intestine	Kidneys Bladder	Liver Gall Bladder	Heart Sm. Intestine	Spleen Stomach	Pericardium Triple Burner

The 3 Hearts – Heart, abdomen, calves: The first heart is the heart in your chest for the oxygenation of the blood. Lower abdominal breathing is considered the second heart for circulation of fluid, Qi and digestion. The third heart is the calf muscles for re-circulation of the blood.

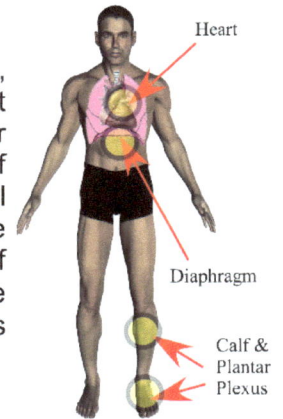

Small Circuit – the linking two energy pathways that run along the midline of the body into a cycling loop. The "fire pathway", Du Mai (Governing Vessel), extends up the back and the other, Ren Mai (Conception Vessel), down the front of the body.

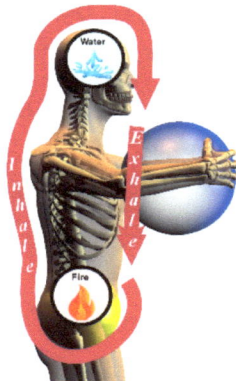

Vessels – there are 8 extraordinary vessels that function as reservoirs of Qi for the Twelve Regular Meridians.

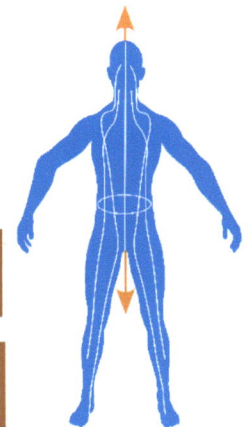

Conception Thrusting Yin Linking Yin Heel	**4 Yin Vessels**
Governing Belt Yang Linking Yang Heel	**4 Yang Vessels**

Taoism - (sometimes Daoism) is a philosophical or ethical tradition of Chinese origin, or faith of Chinese exemplification, that emphasizes living in harmony with the Tao (or Dao). The term Tao means "way", "path", or the "principle".

The Void (Supreme Mystery)

Wuji – ultimate stillness, the beginning of creation.

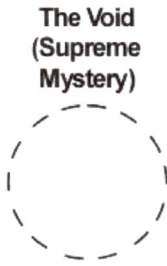

Yang Qi - yang refers to aspects or manifestations of Qi that are relatively positive: Also - immaterial, amorphous, expanding, hollow, light, ascending, hot, dry, warming, bright, aggressive, masculine and active.

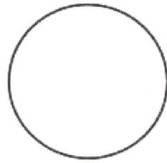

Yin Qi - yin refers to aspects or manifestations of Qi that are relatively negative: Also - material, substantial, condensing, solid, heavy, descending, cold, moist, cooling, dark, female, passive and quiescent.

Taijitu -The term taijitu in modern Chinese is commonly used to mean the simple "divided circle" form (), but it may refer to any of several schematic diagrams that contain at least one circle with an inner pattern of symmetry representing yin and yang.

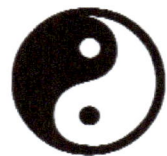

Yi – intellect, manifests as spirit-infused intelligence and understanding.

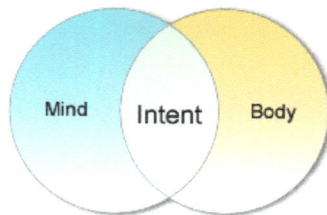

Baihui point - Governing Vessel 20 (GV 20). Sits on the crown of the head.

Jade Pillow – located at the top of the cervical vertebrae (C1).

Great Hammer – located on the midline at the base of the neck, between seventh cervical vertebra and first thoracic vertebra.

Mingmen point – Conception Vessel 6 (CV6), the 'Sea of Qi' located on the lower abdomen.

Qihai point – Conception Vessel 6 (CV6), the 'Sea of Qi' located on the lower abdomen.

Hui Yin point – Conception Vessel 1 (CV1), also known as the base chakra, is located between the genitals and the anus; the part of the body called the perineum.

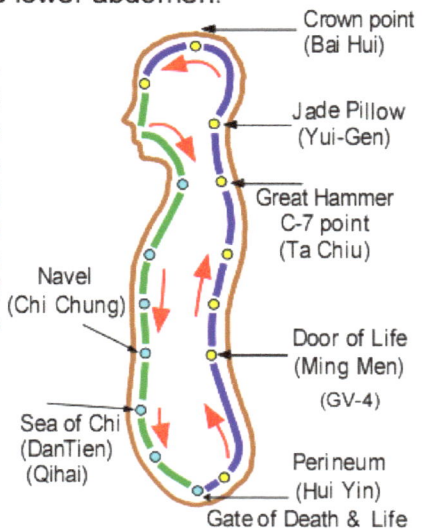

Crown point (Bai Hui)
Jade Pillow (Yui-Gen)
Great Hammer C-7 point (Ta Chiu)
Navel (Chi Chung)
Door of Life (Ming Men) (GV-4)
Sea of Chi (DanTien) (Qihai)
Perineum (Hui Yin)
Gate of Death & Life

Wu Xing or 5 Elements -
The 5 Element theory is a major component of thought within Traditional Chinese Medicine (TCM). Each element represents natural aspects within our world. Natural cycles and interrelationships between these elements, is the basis for this theory. These elements have corresponding relationships within our environment as well as within our own being.

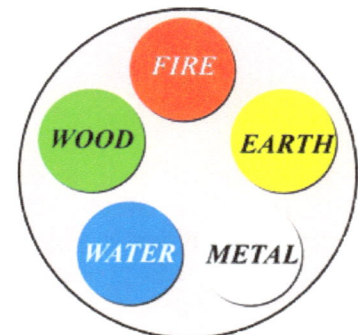

Mind Intent Body

Zang-Fu organs – solid, yin organs are Zang – yang and hollow organs are Fu.

5 Yin Organs
Liver
Heart
Spleen
Lungs
Kidneys

Spleen & Pancreas	Lungs	Kidneys	Liver	Heart

5 Yang Organs
Gall Bladder
Small Intestine
Stomach
Large Intestine
Bladder

Stomach	Large Intestine	Urinary Bladder	Gall Bladder	Small Intestine

FIRE
WOOD
EARTH
WATER METAL

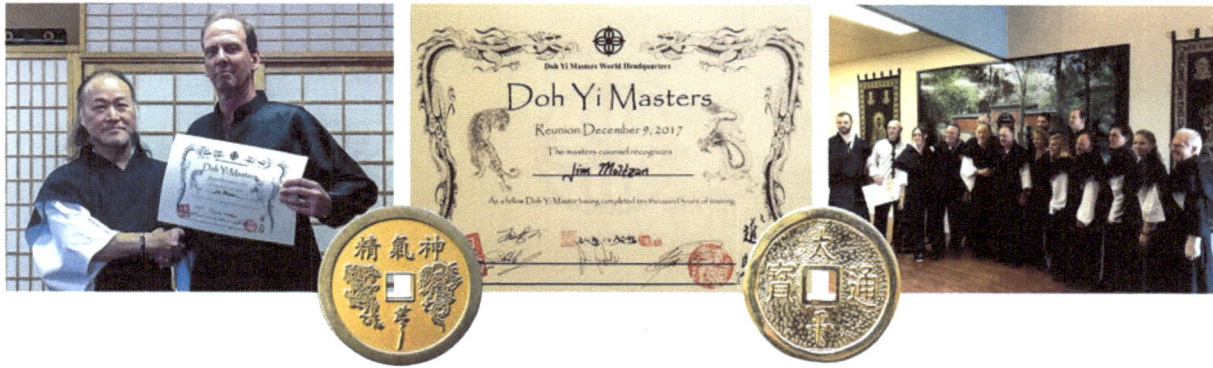

About the Instructor, Author & Artist - Jim Moltzan

My fitness training started at the age of 16 and has continued for almost 45 years. During that time, I attended high school, then college, and worked 2 jobs all while pursuing further training in martial arts and other fitness methods. Many years ago, I started up an additional business to help finance my next goal of owning my own school. I moved to Florida from the Midwest to make this goal a reality. Having owned two wellness and martial arts schools, I have surpassed what I once believed to be my potential. At this stage in my life, I have chosen not to open any more schools, as I found the business aspects took too much focus away from my true passion: training and teaching others.

Beyond my professional endeavors, I am also a husband and father of two grown children. I believe that we must be prepared to work hard mentally, physically and financially to earn our good health and well-being. Not only for ourselves but for our families as well. Good health always comes at a cost whether in time, effort, cost, sacrifice or some combination of the previous.

I returned to college in my later 50's, to pursue my BS in Holistic Health (wellness and alternative medicine). My degree program covered many wide-ranging topics such as anatomy and physiology, meditation, massage, nutrition, herbology, chemistry, biology, history and basis of various medical modalities such as allopathic, Traditional Chinese Medicine, Ayurveda/yoga, naturopathy, chiropractic, and complimentary alternative methods. I also studied religion, mythology of the world, stress relief/management as well as sociology, psychology (human behavior) and cultural issues associated with better health and wellness.

Most of the movements I teach and write about originate from Chinese martial arts. The Qigong (breathing work) is from Chinese Kung Fu and the Korean Dong Han medical Qigong lineage. I have also gained much knowledge of Traditional Chinese Medicine (TCM) from many TCM practitioners, martial arts masters, teachers and peers. This includes many techniques and practices of acupressure (reflexology, auricular, Jing Well, etc.), acupuncture, moxibustion as well as preparation of some herbal remedies and extracts for conditioning and injuries. I have been studying for over 20 years with Zen Wellness, learning medical Qigong as well as other Eastern methods of fitness, philosophy and self-cultivation. I have been recognized as a "Gold Coin" master instructor having trained and taught others for at least 10000 hours or roughly over 35 years. The core fitness movements are from Kung Fu and its forms in Tai Chi, Baguazhang, Dao Yin and Ship Pal Gi (Korean Kung Fu and weapons training). Each martial art has mental, physical and spiritual aspects that can complement and enhance one another. The more ways that you can move your body and engage your mind, the better it is for your overall health.

Physical health, mental well-being and the relationships within our lives; are these the most cherished aspects of our existence? Yet, how much effort do we put towards improving these areas on a daily basis?

Many have used martial arts and other mind-body methods of training as methods of learning to see one's character as others see them. I feel that I can offer the priceless qualities of truth, honor and integrity with my instruction. You must seek the right teacher for you, because in time a student can become similar to their teacher. Through the training that I have experienced and offer to others, an individual can understand and hopefully reach their full potential.

By developing self-discipline to continuously execute and perfect sets of movements, an individual can start to understand not only how they work physically but also mentally and emotionally. You can find your strengths and your weaknesses and improve them both. Through disciplined training, one not only enhances physical abilities but also cultivates mental resilience, allowing them to achieve their fullest potential in all areas of life.

I have co-authored a book, produced numerous other books and journals, graphic charts and study guides related to the mind and body connection and how it relates to martial arts, fitness, and self-improvement. A few hundred of my classes and lectures are viewable on YouTube.com.

Lineage

- o Recognized as a 1000 and 10,000-hour student and teacher

- o Earned gold coins through the Doh Yi Masters and Zen Wellness program

- o Earned a 5th degree in Korean Kung Fu through the Dong Han lineage

Education

Bachelor of Science in Holistic Medicine - Vermont State University

Books Available Through Amazon

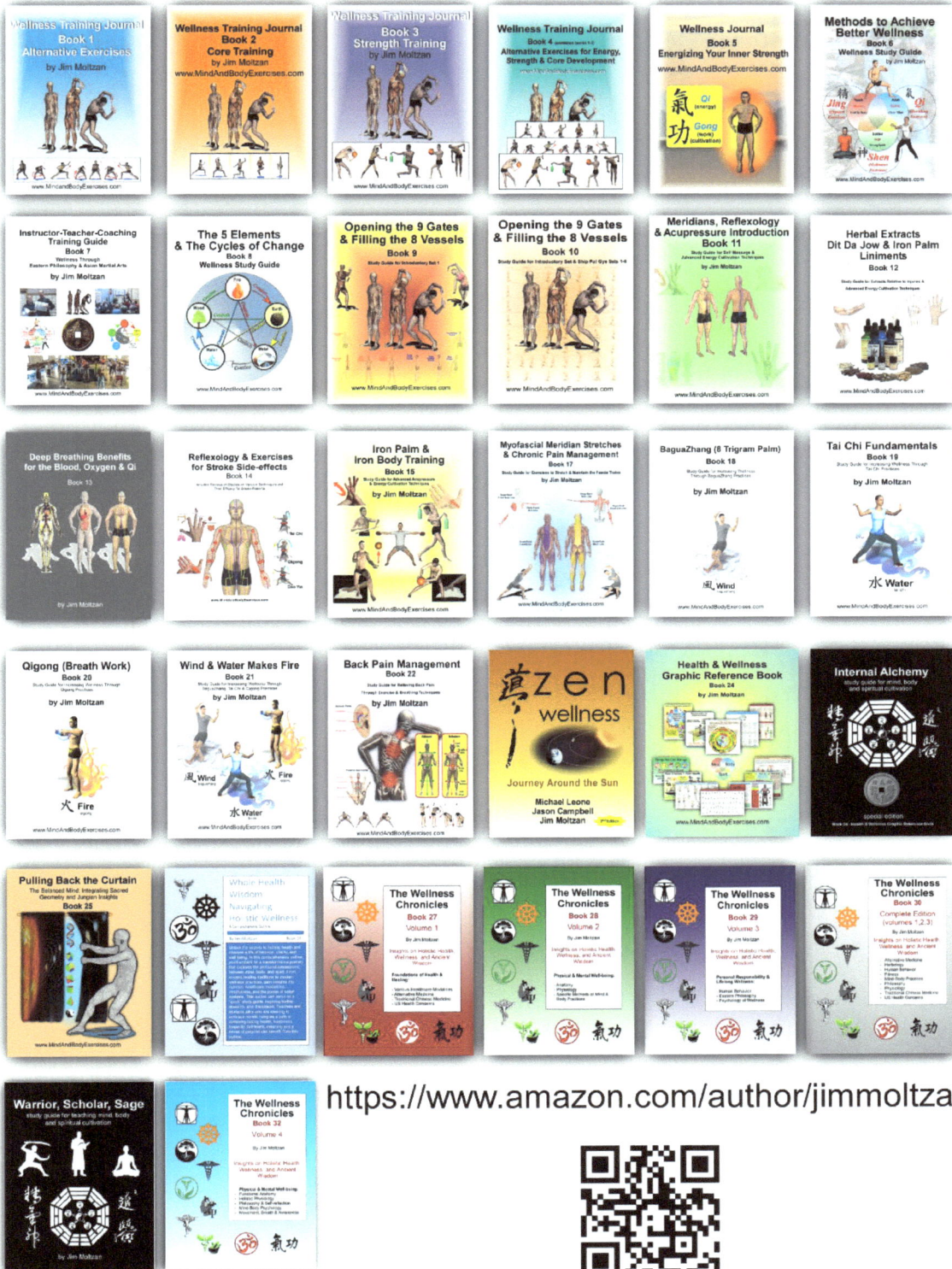

Wellness Training Journal
Book 1
Alternative Exercises
by Jim Moltzan
www.MindandBodyExercises.com

Wellness Training Journal
Book 2
Core Training
by Jim Moltzan
www.MindAndBodyExercises.com

Wellness Training Journal
Book 3
Strength Training
by Jim Moltzan

Wellness Training Journal
Book 4
Alternative Exercises for Energy, Strength & Core Development

Wellness Journal
Book 5
Energizing Your Inner Strength
www.MindAndBodyExercises.com

Methods to Achieve Better Wellness
Book 6
Wellness Study Guide
by Jim Moltzan

Instructor-Teacher-Coaching Training Guide
Book 7
Wellness Through Eastern Philosophy & Asian Martial Arts
by Jim Moltzan

The 5 Elements & The Cycles of Change
Book 8
Wellness Study Guide

Opening the 9 Gates & Filling the 8 Vessels
Book 9
Study Guide for Introductory Set 1

Opening the 9 Gates & Filling the 8 Vessels
Book 10
Study Guide for Introductory Set & Ship Pal Gye Sets 1-4

Meridians, Reflexology & Acupressure Introduction
Book 11
Study Guide for Self Massage & Advanced Energy Cultivation Techniques
by Jim Moltzan

Herbal Extracts
Dit Da Jow & Iron Palm Liniments
Book 12

Deep Breathing Benefits for the Blood, Oxygen & Qi
Book 13
by Jim Moltzan

Reflexology & Exercises for Stroke Side-effects
Book 14

Iron Palm & Iron Body Training
Book 15
by Jim Moltzan

Myofascial Meridian Stretches & Chronic Pain Management
Book 17
by Jim Moltzan

BaguaZhang (8 Trigram Palm)
Book 18
by Jim Moltzan
Wind

Tai Chi Fundamentals
Book 19
by Jim Moltzan
Water

Qigong (Breath Work)
Book 20
by Jim Moltzan
Fire

Wind & Water Makes Fire
Book 21
by Jim Moltzan
Wind   Fire
Water

Back Pain Management
Book 22
by Jim Moltzan

zen wellness
Journey Around the Sun
Michael Leone
Jason Campbell
Jim Moltzan

Health & Wellness Graphic Reference Book
Book 24
by Jim Moltzan

Internal Alchemy
study guide for mind, body and spiritual cultivation
special edition

Pulling Back the Curtain
The Balanced Mind: Integrating Sacred Geometry and Jungian Insights
Book 25
www.MindAndBodyExercises.com

Whole Health Wisdom Navigating Holistic Wellness

The Wellness Chronicles
Book 27
Volume 1
By Jim Moltzan

The Wellness Chronicles
Book 28
Volume 2
By Jim Moltzan

The Wellness Chronicles
Book 29
Volume 3
By Jim Moltzan

The Wellness Chronicles
Book 30
Complete Edition
(volumes 1,2,3)
By Jim Moltzan

Warrior, Scholar, Sage
study guide for teaching mind, body and spiritual cultivation

The Wellness Chronicles
Book 32
Volume 4
By Jim Moltzan

https://www.amazon.com/author/jimmoltzan

Books Titles by Jim Moltzan

Book 1 - Alternative Exercises

Book 2 - Core Training

Book 3 - Strength Training

Book 4 - Combo of 1-3

Book 5 - Energizing Your Inner Strength

Book 6 - Methods to Achieve Better Wellness

Book 7 - Coaching & Instructor Training Guide

Book 8 - The 5 Elements & the Cycles of Change

Book 9 - Opening the 9 Gates & Filling 8 Vessels - Intro Set 1

Book 10 - Opening the 9 Gates & Filling 8 Vessels-sets 1 to 8

Book 11 - Meridians, Reflexology & Acupressure

Book 12 - Herbal Extracts, Dit Da Jow & Iron Palm Liniments

Book 13 - Deep Breathing Benefits for the Blood, Oxygen & Qi

Book 14 - Reflexology for Stroke Side Effects:

Book 15 - Iron Body & Iron Palm

Book 17 - Fascial Train Stretches & Chronic Pain Management

Book 18 - BaguaZhang

Book 19 - Tai Chi Fundamentals

Book 20 - Qigong (breath-work)

Book 21 - Wind & Water Make Fire

Book 22 - Back Pain Management

Book 23 - Journey Around the Sun-2nd Edition

Book 24 - Graphic Reference Book - Internal Alchemy

Book 25 - Pulling Back the Curtain

Book 26 - Whole Health Wisdom: Navigating Holistic Wellness

Book 27 - The Wellness Chronicles (volume 1)

Book 28 - The Wellness Chronicles (volume 2)

Book 29 - The Wellness Chronicles (volume 3)

Book 30 - The Wellness Chronicles (complete edition of 1-3)

On Amazon

Other Products

Laminated Charts 8.5" x 11" or 11" x 17" - over 200 various graphics (check the website)

Qigong - Chi Kung

SKU: ChiKung

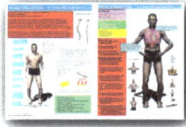

The human body is made up of bones, muscles, and organs amongst other components. Veins, arteries and capillaries carry blood and nutrients throughout to all of the systems and components. Additionally, 12 major energy medians carry the body's energy, "life force" also known as "chi". Ones chi is stored in the lower Dan Tien. Daily emotional imbalances accumulate tension and stress gradually affecting all of the body's systems. Each discomfort, nuisance, irritation or grudge continues to tighten and squeeze the flow of the life force. This is where "dis-ease" claims its foothold.

Strengthen Your Back (set #1)

SKU: StrengthenYourBack1

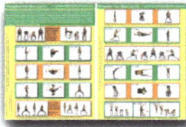

Good health of the lower back starts with good posture. The following set of exercises develop strength and flexibility which improve posture. Strength in the back, hips and abdominals provide a strong cage that houses the internal organs. Flexibility in these areas helps to maintain good blood circulation to the organs and lower body. Lengthening of the spine while exercising reduces stress and tension on the nervous system.

Broadsword 1-10

SKU: Broadsword

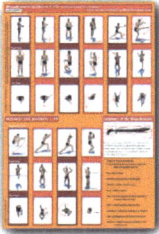

Broadsword training develops the body, mind and spirit well beyond that which can gained from empty hand training alone. The Broadsword has many different sets to be mastered utilizing quick, fluid and precise movements.

Ship Pal Gye set 7 (Kung Fu stance training)

SKU: ShipPalGye7

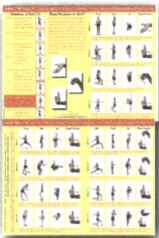

SHIP PAL GYE or Ship Par Gay, is a Korean version of Chinese Shaolin Lohan Qigong, meaning "18 chi movements" or what were supposedly the original 18 drills that Bodhidharma introduced to the Shaolin monks. It is reputed to be the basis for the Shaolin Kung Fu, which in turn, greatly influenced the developments of all branches of Asian fighting arts.

Noble Stances

SKU: NobleStances

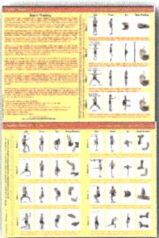

Noble stances are a combination of various stances from different styles of Chinese martial arts. Stances, in this case, meaning correct placement of the feet, knees, hips, and arm positions relative to ones center of gravity. Executing static positions and holding the particular body positions for anyway from a few seconds to several minutes reaps many benefits foremost being able to cultivate a strong and healthy core.

168

Contacts

For more information regarding charts, products, classes and instruction:

www.MindAndBodyExercises.com
info@MindAndBodyExercises.com

www.youtube.com/c/MindandBodyExercises
www.MindAndBodyExercises.wordpress.com

407-234-0119

Social Media:

Facebook: MindAndBodyExercises
Instagram: MindAndBodyExercises
Twitter: MindAndBodyExercise

Jim Moltzan - Mind and Body Exercises
522 Hunt Club Blvd. #305
Apopka, FL 32703

Website

Blog

YouTube
Channel